LOVERS AND LIVERS:
DISEASE CONCEPTS IN HISTORY

Can a disease be an idea? A theory? Does a disease exist without a patient to suffer from it or a medical profession to define it?

In *Lovers and Livers*, Jacalyn Duffin introduces philosophical theories of disease and delves into the history of two distinct afflictions – one old, one new – that serve as examples to show how applying theory can uncover surprising aspects of the medical past and present. Written with humour and compassion, and using poignant examples from Duffin's own clinical experience, *Lovers and Livers* is based on a series of public lectures incorporating audience participation along with a wide variety of sources including art, literature, medical journals, and newspapers.

Duffin's first example of a disease concept – the now possibly defunct disease of lovesickness – had its origins in the poetry of antiquity and its demise in twentieth-century scepticism, but Duffin argues that it may not be as *passé* as is generally thought. The second example is the newer disease hepatitis C. Duffin demonstrates that it too stems from ancient tradition and that it has been shaped by discoveries in virology and recent tragedies in transfusion medicine, as well as by legislators, journalists, and patients.

Providing a lively overview of ideas surrounding disease, *Lovers and Livers* will appeal to scholars of history, philosophy, and medicine, as well as to the general reader.

(The Joanne Goodman Lectures)

JACALYN DUFFIN is a professor in the Faculty of Health Sciences, the Department of History, and the Department of Philosophy, and holds the Hannah Chair in the History of Medicine at Queen's University.

Lovers and Livers

Disease Concepts in History

The 2002 Joanne Goodman Lectures

JACALYN DUFFIN

UNIVERSITY OF TORONTO PRESS
Toronto Buffalo London

© University of Toronto Press Incorporated 2005
Toronto Buffalo London
Printed in Canada

ISBN 0-8020-3868-9 (cloth)
ISBN 0-8020-3805-0 (paper)

Printed on acid-free paper

Library and Archives Canada Cataloguing in Publication

Duffin, Jacalyn
   Lovers and livers : disease concepts in history / Jacalyn Duffin.

(The 2002 Joanne Goodman lectures)
Includes bibliographical references and index.
ISBN 0-8020-3868-9 (bound)   ISBN 0-8020-3805-0 (pbk.)

1. Diseases – Social aspects.   2. Lovesickness.   3. Hepatitis C.
4. Medicine – Philosophy.   I. Title.   II. Series: Joanne Goodman
lectures ; 2002.
RB151.D83 2005   610'.1   C2004-907256-0

University of Toronto Press acknowledges the financial assistance to
its publishing program of the Canada Council for the Arts and the
Ontario Arts Council.

University of Toronto Press acknowledges the financial support for
its publishing activities of the Government of Canada through the
Book Publishing Industry Development Program (BPIDP).

The Joanne Goodman Lecture Series

has been established by Joanne's family

and friends to perpetuate the memory of her

blithe spirit, her quest for knowledge, and

the rewarding years she spent at the

University of Western Ontario.

To the memory of

Mirko Drazen Grmek

Contents

Tables and Figures

Illustrations

Acknowledgments

These lectures were written in France and Italy during a sabbatical leave granted by Queen's University and supported by Associated Medical Services/Hannah Institute. Now that they are complete, I realize that I had been 'working on' disease ideas (without writing about them) for most of my life as a historian and a teacher. To have the opportunity to address a wide audience on this subject was a welcome challenge and a tremendous privilege.

The fascination of disease concepts was the gift of my late mentor, Mirko Drazen Grmek, who supervised my doctorate in Paris. For two decades, this interest has been sharpened and nurtured by the provocative questions of my students in philosophy, history, and medicine at the University of Ottawa and Queen's University. Many others helped enthusiastically with the research and writing; they read and shredded chapters with gusto, supplied information with patience, and doled out inspiration by example. They include Maung T. (Bertie) Aye, Ron Batt, Morris Blajchman, K. Codell Carter, Henry Dinsdale, Dale Dotten, Monika Dutt, Toby Gelfand, Martin French, Ross Kilpatrick, Horace Krever, Ray Matthews, Adam D. McDonald, Peter and Hilary Neary, Michael Orsini, Patricia Peppin, Paul Potter, Neville Thompson, and the tireless staff of Bracken

Health Sciences Library. My work at home and abroad was facilitated in many ways by kind friends and family, especially Thomas W. Dukes, Elsbeth Heaman, Terrie Romano, Robert David Wolfe, and Cherrilyn Yalin.

I am grateful to Eddie Goodman and his family for their generosity in establishing this lecture series that celebrates the life and commemorates the tragic passing of a young woman who loved learning and her alma mater. Humbled by the list of my distinguished predecessors, I am especially indebted to the committee for selecting me as a speaker. And I thank the members of the Goodman audience – some of whom turned out faithfully three days in a row – for their penetrating questions and willing participation in the games, experiments, and homework. In this book, may they find good memories of our shared evenings and a fair accounting of their contributions, together with my gratitude.

Abbreviations

ALT	alanine aminotransferase
CMAJ	*Canadian Medical Association Journal*
DSM	*Diagnostic and Statistical Manual*
HCV	hepatitis C virus
HIV	human immunodeficiency virus
JAMA	*Journal of the American Medical Association*
MRI	magnetic resonance imaging
OCD	obsessive-compulsive disorder
PET	positron emission tomography
PMS	premenstrual syndrome
PRV	polycythemia rubra vera
SARS	severe acute respiratory syndrome
SIDS	sudden infant death syndrome
STD	sexually transmitted disease
VD	venereal disease

1

The Disease Game: An Introduction to the Concepts and Construction of Disease

In these pages I will try to convince you that diseases are ideas. You may think of them as scientific puzzles, or as frightening scourges, or as slow, painful torments. I do not want to dissuade you from those views, but I hope you will also see how they can be ideas influenced by the tastes and preoccupations of society. The history of disease, then, is an exercise in intellectual history, intimately related to culture and philosophy of knowledge in any time or place.

In this first chapter, we will examine general *definitions* of disease, looking for what characteristics are common to all diseases. In each of the next two chapters, we will look at specific examples: first, an old disease that seems to have vanished (lovesickness), and second, a new disease that has appeared within my career (hepatitis C). In investigating these two histories of a defunct disease and of a novel disease, I will apply the basic principles described in this chapter; the theories are useful tools of analysis that allow us to uncover some surprising things about how we decide what is sickness and what is not. These three chapters correspond to the Joanne Goodman lectures read at the University of Western Ontario on three consecutive evenings in October 2002. Members of the audience willingly participated in games, homework, and quizzes each day; their contributions are included here too.

For some time now, historians and philosophers have explored disease concepts. I rely on the work of many predecessors, including Georges Canguilhem, Ludwik Fleck, Michel Foucault, Lester King, Oswei Temkin, Robert Hudson, Guenter Risse, Charles Rosenberg, Susan Sontag, K. Codell Carter, Annemarie Mol, and, above all, my mentor, Mirko Drazen Grmek.[1] My only claim to originality in this first chapter is in the heuristic approach to explaining the problem.

Audience Participation: The Disease Game

To break the ice at the first lecture, I asked the audience to participate in what I call 'the disease game,' a simple exercise in word association. I have been using this device in my undergraduate philosophy classes and other places since 1989. I say eight disease words, slowly, writing them on the board at the front of the lecture hall. On a slip of paper that had been distributed when they arrived, the people in the audience jot down the first word or phrase that comes to mind on hearing each word. After the eight word associations are complete, the audience is invited to the front to transcribe their responses on the blackboard under the appropriate headings. In London, October 2002, the slips of paper were collected at the end of the lecture, and all the responses appear in table 1.1.

Few of us have ever seen a case of leprosy, plague, or smallpox. But the disease game shows that even if we have never seen someone suffering from these conditions, we certainly have ideas about them. Furthermore, our ideas converge – several people chose identical or closely related words. Cancer was associated with the word 'death' twenty times; tuberculosis with 'lung(s)' eleven times; headache with 'pain' twenty-two times. Were we to collect all the words associated with each disease and use them in a little essay, we would probably come up with a fair approximation of the concept of that one disease held collectively by an academic subset of the citizens of London, Ontario, Canada, in October 2002.

What Is a Disease Concept?

The word associations sparked by each disease tend to converge, but different diseases provoke a wide array of responses. In the fifteen years I have played this game with various audiences, leprosy nearly always inspires thoughts of the Bible; smallpox, of children. Even when the similarities of two conditions are great, disease ideas will differ from one another; they have personalities. For example, smallpox and leprosy are both infectious conditions of the skin; one has vanished, the other is rare. We might expect that they would evoke similar associations; however, they do not. Our ultimate goal in this chapter is to find what all diseases have in common, but first we will dwell on the ways in which they differ, as shown by the responses in table 1.1.

One distinction between the different disease concepts is prompted by our distance from, or familiarity with, the problems. The first reaction is subjective, triggered by a personal recollection. Look how often responses to the word 'headache' emphasize pain. Who has never had a headache? No one. The experience of tuberculosis and leprosy may be just as painful, but the audience was less familiar with those conditions. Similarly, the all-too-common and disturbing disease of cancer provoked thoughts of suffering and the names of loved ones who struggle with it. If we 'know' the disease, our reactions are empathic and sensory, rather than detached.

Speakers of English can separate thoughts on the matter of subjectivity and objectivity by establishing a linguistic convention between 'illness' and 'disease.' 'Illness,' on the one hand, applies to the subjective aspects of suffering, the problem experienced by the individual patient. In medical parlance, features of the illness are commonly called symptoms – they are felt by the sufferer. 'Disease,' on the other hand, represents our ideas about that illness. The words 'disease' and 'illness' are used interchangeably by doctors, scientists, and the general public. I have no illusions about changing that widespread habit. But for the purposes of this book, I adhere to this distinction, which a long line of philosophers and historians have found helpful.

In general, illnesses change slowly – the constancy of human suffering is a medical *longue durée*. The human organism has always suffered from pain, swelling, thirst, hunger, anorexia, sneezing, cough, trouble breathing, fainting, fever, sweating, nausea, vomiting, diarrhea, bleeding, loss of movement or sen-

Table 1.1 'Disease Game' word association, London, Ontario, October 2002

Plague	Leprosy	Headache	Cancer
14th century	Africa × 2	Advil	20th century
Athens	armadillo	alcohol	big C
awful	bell	aneurysm	black
black × 8	Ben Hur × 3	aspirin × 10	blood × 2
black death × 6	Bible × 4	bad	breast
bubonic × 9	biblical	brain	brother
death × 6	body parts	dean	cell(s) × 4
disease × 5	books	drug	chemo × 4
dog	chronic	exams	chronic
epidemiology	colony × 2	head	chronicity
Europe	David and Peter	hell	colon
fatal	disease × 5	hurts	crab × 3
fleas	disfigurement × 2	hypertension	cure
* game(s) × 5	exile × 3	Laura	deadly
god	face-off	medicine	death × 20
* ground	foul	menstruation × 2	destructive
horror	frog	migraine × 5	die
houses	gross	Mom	disease
illness	hand	mother	growth × 3
itch	Hansen	Motrin	horrible
mass death	Hawaii	nuisance	is there a cure?
Middle Ages × 2	horrid	owwwwa	lungs
moby	illness × 2	pain × 22	medicine
night	India × 2	pill	mother
*playground	isolation	rarely	nuclear
rats × 4	Jerusalem	sleep	often
ring a rosy	Jesus	soreness	pain
*school yard	Lazarus	stress × 3	personal
scourge	leopard	term papers	radiation
Shakespeare	limbs × 2	throb	research
smallpox	lions	tumour	scary
spread	mendicant	Tylenol × 6	sister
sweep	numb	wife	smoking
tennis	plague		society
Thucydides	Robert the Bruce		therapy
VD	rot × 2		tiger
vermin	rotting × 2		tough
yuck	scab		tragic
	scars		treatment
* several heard me	Schweitzer		tropic
say 'play'	sick		tumour × 2
	skin × 3		unsolved
	skin disease		web
	sore		women
	sores		
	spots		
	Teresa		
	terrible		
	third world		
	unclean		
	white		
	withering		
	yuck		

Table 1.1, *continued*

PMS	AIDS	Smallpox	Tuberculosis
45	Africa × 10	again?	Bethune
anger	chimp	blankets	breathing
annoyance × 2	chocolate	blisters	chest
annoying	communicable	board	chest X-ray
argh	disease	Catherine the Great	Chopin
bitch	deadly × 3	chicken pox × 3	coal miner
bloating	death × 4	childhood	consumption
blood	disease	children × 2	consumptive 19th-
cranky	drugs	conquest	century writers
disability	dying	cowpox	contagious
emotion	end	deadly	cough × 8
fake	end of 20th century	death × 2	cows
forever	epidemic	disfiguration	CXR[ay]
girl	gay	eradicated × 3	disease × 2
girlfriend	gays	Europe	Doc Holliday
grumpy	Grmek	extinct	easily transmitted
hard	help	fear	hospital × 2
headache	helps	First Nations	intravenous
hell	herpes	gone?	is it coming back?
hormones	HIV × 5	immunity	lung(s) × 11
horse	homosexual	inoculation scar	Madame Bovary
hot flashes	homosexuality	itch	romantics
irritating	homosexuals	kids	miliary
irritation	horrible	lesions	mountains
misery	ignorance	little box	Norman Bethune
mood × 2	infection	long time ago	old
mood changes	modern	Middle Ages	penicillin
mood swings	modern world	Montreal × 2	person who died of
moods	monkey	Mozart	plague
mother	needle	native Americans × 2	poverty × 2
myth	New York	native peoples	red
nerves	pill	natives × 2	returning
no	problems	old × 2	sanatorium × 7
no HRT	sad	pustules	sister
not me	savage	pox scars	South American
overrated	scandal	quarantine	countries
pain × 4	scary	red	still around
pain in the neck	scourge	scabs	test
period	sex × 4	scars × 4	vaccine × 2
post mens.	sexual transmission	scary	Victorian London
premenstrual	sod	scourge	virus
syndrome	sorrow	Simpsons	wasting × 2
real?	syringe	skin	white
roommate	terrible	Somalia	white plague
sucks	thin	spots × 3	worms
syndrome	third world	vaccination × 4	Zauberberg
tension	tragedy	vaccine × 7	
tragic	tragic × 2	virus	
trials	virus	wiped out	
what is it?	wasting × 2		
wife × 3			
women × 17			

sation, and sudden death – and various combinations of them. They are the 'symptoms' or complaints (for their relationship to 'signs,' see page 19). The constellations or patterns of symptoms can change through time with ecological shifts, owing to natural or human intervention. Grmek invented the term 'pathocenosis' to refer to the set of diseases or ailments that affect a population in a given time and space.[2] When one disease drops out, another may come along to take its place.

What changes far more quickly through time, place, and culture is how people talk about these various illnesses and what ideas they construct to account for them. *That* is the disease. Of course, the concept of disease incorporates an understanding of the illness, and sometimes the formulations of diseases are strongly shaped by the distinctive manifestations of exemplary ailments.[3] But a disease concept contains much more than the symptoms of the illness.

The sufferer (or patient) is also part of the disease idea. Cancer and AIDS bring to our minds the names of people who have had these diseases. And for PMS (premenstrual syndrome), the responses seem to indicate that only half of the audience could ever have experienced it personally – the other half is aware of it, but perhaps not too inclined to take it seriously. Many wrote words that identified the imagined sufferer: bitch, girl, girlfriend, mother, wife, woman/women. A person who played the disease game responded to PMS with the words 'Not Me.'

At this point, we can say that a disease concept blends ideas about the illness and ideas about the people who are likely to suffer from it. With little effort we could make many of the disease game responses fit into either 'illness' or 'patient.' The leftover words are also interesting.

More than a description of symptoms and patients, however, a disease is also an explanation, or even a little *theory* about an illness. Not only must the disease change to keep up with new observations of sickness and new science, it must change to keep up with what is considered appropriate in terms of philosophy of knowledge (epistemology). The rules that govern clear thinking will also govern disease ideas, just as much as they shape beliefs in logic, biology, physics, and justice. Now I will expand on this notion using historical examples, which appear 'out of order.' Chronology is not my purpose.

Reducing Disease to Its Component Parts

Sometimes the illness dominates a disease concept. In the seventeenth and eighteenth centuries, philosophy self-consciously placed high value on the senses as the source of knowledge in a tradition that came to be known as 'sensualist' philosophy. Its proponents included John Locke (1632–1704) and Etienne Bonnot, Abbé de Condillac (1714–80). At that time, a number of 'new' diseases were identified through careful observation of the patients' symptoms, their duration, sequence, pattern, and combination. Conditions formerly thought to be one disease suddenly became two or more diseases as judged by subtle variations in symptoms.[4] In the classic descriptions by Thomas Sydenham (1624–89) of gout, chorea, scarlet fever, and measles, the manifestations of the patient's suffering loom large. Medical authors who embraced this 'sensualist' philosophy called themselves 'nosologists,' those who write about diseases. Doctors became adept at reading 'signs' embedded in the various symptoms and their sequence in order to diagnose the problem (see page 19). These illness-dominated diseases were constellations of symptoms, classified into family trees by orders, genera, and species. During early modern times, one could not be sick without feeling sick.

Some diseases are still classified and identified in this symptom-based way, especially those of unknown cause: for example, fevers that appear to be contagious; lymphomas and other malignancies; or mental disorders that are described (and classified) in the successive editions of the *Diagnostic and Statistical Manual (DSM).*[5]

In the disease game (table 1.1), the illness aspect of the disease concept is evident in those responses that emphasize symptoms of the disease: pain for headache; scabs, scars, and skin lesions for leprosy or smallpox; lungs and coughing for tuberculosis.

Still working from our word associations, we can find other broad categories common to all diseases. The rubrics in table 1.2 are the anatomical parts of a well-dressed disease concept. They provide a framework for beginning to investigate any disease concept in the present or in the past. If you look in any medical text from just about any era, information about diseases will follow some or all of these categories. Not all aspects of a disease idea will be addressed in every concept; sometimes, one or another category may be ignored.

Table 1.2 Components of a well-dressed disease concept

Illness (or Symptoms)	what the suffering is like characteristics of the problem
Patients	who suffers from it demographics and epidemiology
Name (Diagnosis)	what we call it
Outcome (Prognosis)	what will happen
Cause	what we think provokes it
Treatment or prevention	what we do to make it go away

One major component of the disease concept is still missing from the list in table 1.2. It is missing in most of the medical books, too. So important and so pervasive is this component that it is nearly impossible to see. We will return to it shortly. The audience had to wait for it, but the impatient reader may sneak a peek at page 21. More sanguine readers can think about what it might be while we explore how each of these new categories interacts with the overriding disease concept.

Disease Names (Diagnosis)

A name or diagnosis is crucial. It provides a label, an identity, an organizing principle for further discussion. Usually a disease concept is born with its first name, although the associated illness may have been recognized long before. Having been named, a disease takes on a distinct life of its own, separate from other diseases.[6] Historically, names reveal presumed causes, presumed manifestations, presumed discoverers, or presumed patients. Take, for example, the early names for European syphilis. Thought to have been brought from the Americas with the return of Christopher Columbus, syphilis first made an appearance during the late-fifteenth-century siege of Naples by the French army and its Spanish mercenaries. New to Europe, this disease was variously called the 'French disease' by the Italians, the 'English disease' and the 'Spanish disease' by the French, and the 'Neopolitan disease' by the Spaniards. It was also called the 'great pox,' in recognition of its first symptom of a large, blister-like chancre. Xenophobic suspicions were compounded, as euphemism was piled upon euphemism: lues (Latin for 'plague' or 'pest'); 'syphilis' based on the name of the sinning shepherd in the sixteenth-century allegorical poem by Girolamo Fracastoro (1478?–1553); and modern acronyms, including VD and STD.[7]

Similarly, the multiple names for AIDS in its early history spoke with grim cynicism of anticipated sufferers as well as the illness – 'GRID' (for gay-related immunodeficiency), '4-H-disease' (referring to the anticipated patients: Haitians, hemophiliacs, homosexuals, and heroin users).[8] Patients are also remembered explicitly in disease names, such as Christmas disease (for Factor IX deficiency) or Lou Gehrig's disease (for motor neuron disease, also called amyotrophic lateral sclerosis, or ALS).

Other disease names describe symptoms. The name 'gout,' or in French 'goutte' – a 'drop' or a 'dripping' – was related to dropsy, which was thought to be caused by a liquid distilled drop by drop on the joint. Gout was also called 'podagra' or 'podalgia' from Greek words for 'foot' and 'seizure' or 'pain.' In the eighteenth century, when doctors were avidly identifying diseases by their symptoms, various descriptive names were commonplace, many of them hangovers from antiquity. For example, periodic fevers – tertian, quartan, etc. – described the cycles of fever and chills that characterized what is now malaria. 'Malaria' itself speaks of the 'bad air' (or 'miasma') that was suspected of causing the disease, just as its French word, 'paludisme,' reminds us of marshes where miasmata abound (with mosquitoes). Croup and whooping cough are onomato-poeic names for childhood respiratory ailments. Scarlatina, rou-geola (measles), smallpox, and yaws (from French 'framboises') describe the skin changes that typify them. In fact, many skin diseases today are known by Latinized descriptions of the typi-cal appearance: pityriasis rosea, acne rosacea, lichen planus, erythreme multiforme, tinea pedis, and rhinophyma. If you rec-ognize it and remember a little Latin, you can be a diagnostic whiz in dermatology!

Disease names can change often. When researching medical history of the recent past, a useful trick is to look at the year when the disease name first appeared in the *Index Medicus* or as a medical subject (MeSH) heading in *Medline*, which is the com-prehensive, computerized database of medical literature. That year will not necessarily correspond to the original description, but it will indicate a moment when the disease reached a state of conventional recognition. Throughout my career as a physician, several new disease names were added: for example, Legion-naires' disease (1979) and West Nile fever (1991) – named for likely patients and place; toxic shock (1968), post-traumatic stress disorder (1981), AIDS (1983), attention deficit disorder (1984), BSE (1992), and, soon after these lectures, SARS (2003) – all named for their symptoms or signs.

Prognosis

In certain periods or places, prognosis (or knowledge of the outcome) was much more important than the diagnosis. In antiquity, the credibility of physicians and priests resided in the accuracy of their predictions. Diseases were spoken of simply and nonspecifically as disease, pestilence, or plague. The task was to identify those people who would die and those who would live. Careful physicians declined to treat conditions that were fatal – not only for their patients' comfort but for their own job security. The death of a patient on treatment would reflect badly on her doctor's skill.

Today prognosis is expressed in terms of statistics and survival rates. We try to determine a fair estimation of how many out of one hundred people with exactly the same diagnosis and extent of illness will live for two years or five years or recover completely. Prognosis also drives legal concerns to define and construct disease: a person who dies too soon, or who suffers more or for longer than she 'ought to' have suffered, may be in a position to claim compensation if fault is proved on the part of another.[9]

Causes

The categories of perceived prognosis, cause, and treatment vary more than other categories through time. A new disease is often created when one or more of these components is reconsidered and replaced. Historians who are interested in change will focus on them; the medically trained like to call it 'progress,' and maybe it is. A naive or 'Whiggish' form of disease history describes the past as if it were merely a search for the cause or treatment that we now accept. A more sophisticated disease history would study the perceived causes and treatments in the context of time and place; it would also give special attention to stability of concepts and the reasons why what seems 'wrong' now once seemed 'right' back then. Causes and treatments must correspond to what is philosophically and scientifically reasonable.

At any given time, many well-defined diseases have no known cause or treatment, although hypotheses may abound. Correct or erroneous by current standards, those hypotheses reveal the cultural and scientific priorities of the time in which they emerged. Disease concepts relate illness to ideas about how the world works. In religious cultures, the disease concept connects illness to the will of a deity. In more secular cultures, explanations are sought in the material world. For example, in distant antiquity, epilepsy was called 'the sacred disease' because it was thought to be caused by a god. A Hippocratic author of about the fifth century BC disputed that idea and argued that the sacred disease was no more or less divine than any other: it was the result of phlegm blocking the passage of air through the vessels to the brain.[10] In this case, the Hippocratic writer took the account of the illness out of one paradigm – a religious worldview – to place it in another – a material view of the four bodily structures and fluids (humours).

The perceived cause of a disease could be more important than its manifestations when it came to finding a diagnosis or a treatment. To illustrate this possibility let us return to the example of disease sent by a deity. In the *Iliad*, Homer sang of a great 'pestilence' (with no other specific name), sent by Apollo to punish the Greeks for Agamemnon's refusal to accept the proffered ransom and return Chryseis to her father, his priest. The symptoms of the pestilence are barely described: it affected many people and led to death. It was more important to this religious society to determine the divine cause: a soothsayer revealed Agamemnon's guilt. The daughter was restored to her father, penitent offerings were made, and the disease went away. All the Greeks were held responsible for the behaviour of their chief. That is an example of disease as punishment.

Similar stories of punishment are told in the Old Testament of the Bible: for example, the plagues of Egypt sent to help Moses liberate the Hebrew slaves (Exodus 9 and 11–12), and deaths of Assyrians who were slayed by an angel because their king planned to destroy Jerusalem (2 Kings 19.35).

God-sent disease also occurred in the form of a test. Thus, long-suffering Job endured forty-two biblical chapters of grotesque misery, tenaciously refusing to curse his God. Forbearance was the correct response to this suffering; it was the correct 'treatment,' because, in the end, Job recovered all his losses: family, wealth, and health. Thus, we speak of people who endure long illnesses as having the patience of Job.

Causes of disease reveal political and philosophical perspectives. For fourteenth-century bubonic plague, various causes were mooted about by different contemporary commentators: food, water, weather, other people (especially strangers and enemies), the astronomical conjunction of planets, the dissolute practices of the clergy, and a surfeit of Jews, witches, and village idiots (take your choice). Each presumed cause inspired a therapeutic response. Several causes and several types of causes for one disease were readily tolerated by physicians until even a century ago, when they were challenged, if not overthrown, by bacteriology and the rise of germ theory. In his recent book, philosopher K. Codell Carter contends that the rise of causal concepts for all diseases that favour unique, universal, and specific causes is a product of philosophical as well as medical changes in the last century and a half.[11]

The discovery of a new cause sometimes creates two or more diseases out of one. Hemophilia provides a good example. The tendency to bleed was known to be inherited from mother to son since at least Talmudic antiquity. By the twentieth century, however, bleeding was divided and subdivided into many different diseases. Classical hemophilia is now considered a functional absence of a protein that helps blood to clot, called factor VIII.[12] A new clotting factor is found only when someone who *lacks* it comes to researchers' attention and is investigated. Hemophilia, Christmas disease, and Von Willebrand's disease are different bleeding disorders characterized by inherited deficiencies of one or more of the clotting factors. Other bleeders have inherited problems of the platelet cells that promote clots: weak platelets of various sizes and shapes have been sorted into Bernard-Soulier disease, Glanzman's thromboasthenia, and Wiskott Aldrich syndrome. Certain of these conditions have additional, otherwise insignificant, traits that help in diagnosis: for example, people with Wiskott Aldrich platelets sometimes have eczema of the skin. These subtle variations are welcomed by astute clinicians who keep up in science and love the elegance of the diagnostic dance.[13]

A change in cause does not have to create a new disease, although it may bring new treatments. During my career, peptic ulcer disease has had several different 'causes' and 'treatments,' but it did not vanish. First, it was an anatomical condition, a little bleeding crater in the stomach or intestine that required surgery, such as subtotal gastrectomy, pyloroplasty, and the cutting of the vagus nerve. Next, it was caused by hyperacidity and linked to the patient's stress level and personality type. Treatment was diet, milk, antacids, and psychotherapy. Then, it became an immunochemical disorder treated by blocking histamine-II receptors with cimetidine, a Nobel prize–winning drug. Then, with the discovery of the bacterium *helicobacter pylori*, it became an infection to be treated with antibiotics.[14] A vibrant etiological history for a single disease in such a short time!

Treatment

Just as a new cause can create a new disease, new treatments can do the same. In the early sixteenth century, Fracastoro wrote his treatise on the French disease (syphilis) to promote mercury as a cure. His work is remembered for the allegorical poem that gave the disease its name (and its start), rather than for his recommended therapy, which is now considered a poison. Yet it was his confidence in the effectiveness of mercury that had motivated him to describe the disease.

Another example of therapy creating disease comes from the foxglove leaf (or digitalis). Brought from folk medicine into medical orthodoxy in the late eighteenth century, foxglove worked well for some people with dropsy or swelling, but not for others. Its proponents thought of it as a diuretic that increased urination. But the new treatment created a previously unappreciated distinction in dropsies: those that responded were one disease (later attributed to heart failure); and those that did not were another (later attributed to kidney failure, lymphatic blockage, or venous stasis). Digitalis is still considered effective for swollen legs and wet lungs, but only if they are thought to be caused by a failing heart.

Operations are treatments too. The advent of anesthesia and antisepsis in the mid-nineteenth century meant not only that surgical procedures could be performed safely and painlessly, they could also be imagined as plausible solutions to anatomical problems. The *possibility* of an operation to remove an inflamed appendix advanced the concept of appendicitis. It moved from a vague condition, known for less than a hundred years as localized peritonitis or 'perityphilitis,' to a well-known and widely feared diagnosis.[15] Similarly, the *possibility* of surgery to tighten up the sagging organs of aging bellies was instrumental in creating the 'new disease,' visceroptosis (or droopy gut syndrome). Many stomachs were opened to relieve the back pain that was said to characterize visceroptosis. Publishing on the subject increased in each year during the first half of the twentieth century and then waned, twice, while surgeons engaged in war work. The disease no longer exists, although we retain its memory in procedures to resuspend individual organs such as kidney and uterus.[16]

Sometimes diseases are created deliberately to provide a commercial market. One can think of the patent remedies of the late nineteenth century that exploited the widespread weariness of women to sell Lydia Pinkham's pink pills for pale people. Recently, the pharmaceutical industry has promoted disease creation to increase profits and consumer demand. Prozac was so well publicized by its makers that people who were not depressed clamoured to use it as a personality enhancer for socially demanding situations, such as dating and job interviews.[17] The advent of osteoporosis as an epidemic has been prompted by industrial-scale promotion of what is peculiarly called 'hormone replacement therapy' (or HRT).[18] Whatever the benefits may be for thinning bone, one thing is certain: the medication does not really *replace* hormones; it raises them to levels that are unnaturally high for the older age group. Even more blatant disease creation followed the introduction of Viagra. With the help of a famous and brave American senator, Robert Dole, Pfizer created a public information campaign that unleashed a lucrative epidemic of 'erectile dysfunction' (called ED by those in the know). The word 'impotence,' implying powerlessness or weakness, just had to go. With a more socially acceptable name, and a respectable male who was macho enough to emulate, the drug became a bestseller before it was released. And ED became another disease caused, in part, by its treatment.[19]

Following hard upon the success of Viagra, the pharmaceutical industry seems to be playing a key role in the complex definition of female sexual dysfunction. Treatments construct diseases. From 1997, several conferences have been held with drug company involvement in an effort to define the problem and to draw attention to it. This conscious building of a new disease to satisfy commercial ambitions advances steadily notwithstanding resistance and criticism in the medical literature.[20]

Diseases without Symptoms: The Power of Signs

Diseases do not have to have symptoms. In other words, a disease can exist without illness. For example, high blood pressure usually has no symptoms at all; yet, it is a 'real' disease for which the taxpayer pays a lot of money to keep seniors stocked in anti-hypertensive medications. The same might be said for cancers of the breast, prostate, or cervix, all now diagnosed by the special government-sponsored screening tests of mammography, PSA (prostate specific antigen), and PAP (Papanicoulou) smears. Symptomless high blood pressure or occult cancer have much higher status as diseases than does chronic fatigue syndrome (CFS) – a condition laden with a baffling mixture of bothersome symptoms.[21] What does hyptertension have that CFS does not? Signs.

Semiotics (or semiology) was embraced by literary criticism in the 1950s; however, medics have been reading signs in their patients' stories and appearance for more than two thousand years.[22] Signs are objective indicators of a problem that are detectable to an outsider. Like the signs on the highway, they point to either a diagnosis or a prognosis. The distinction between symptom and sign is the difference between what is subjective (felt by the patient) and what is objective (visible to the observer). Sometimes extra knowledge can turn a simple symptom or set of symptoms into a sign. For example, a patient describes a chest pain that squeezes under the breastbone, radiates down the left arm and into the neck, comes on with exercise, and subsides with rest. *With a little knowledge*, a doctor, a medical student, or a lay person will recognize this symptom as a sign of heart disease. The Hippocratic writings include many signs of disease that are of this type: symptoms (or a sequence of symptoms) imbued with meaning by prior knowledge become signs.[23] But in every era, knowledge of the available disease categories is essential for symptoms to be understood as signs. Expressed mathematically, symptom + knowledge = sign.

But I hasten to add that not all signs are symptoms perceived by the patient. Signs can also be characteristics of the illness that the observer seeks and finds without the patient being aware. Reading a *diagnosis* rather than a prognosis from the patient's pulse, respiration, or urine was established at least by the time of Galen in the second century AD (see chapter 2). The practice of reading pulses was extended as a more focused diagnostic project in the Middle Ages and early modern period.[24] With the advent of scientific positivism in the early nineteenth century, greater emphasis was placed on the measurable observations of physicians than on patient perception. For example, the stethoscope was used to detect fatal tuberculosis in the chests of people who felt completely well. Clinical medicine developed an extensive vocabulary of elegant signs: enlarged lymph nodes, tiny hemorrhages in the back of an eye, a trace of jaundice, an absent reflex, a wide pulse pressure, an altered blood test. Some signs, like those generated by percussion, will bear the names of the manoeuvres required to elicit them, such as 'shifting dullness'; others, such as dullness over Traube's space and Skodiac resonance, bear the names of their discoverers. By 1900, the patient no longer had the final word on whether or not she was sick. In contrast to the illness-based disease concepts of the eighteenth century and earlier, one no longer had to feel sick to be sick.[25]

The twentieth century saw the advent of a host of new signs. Physicians working on a diagnosis could move from eyeing, sniffing, and tasting urine, to heating it in a spoon, to looking at it under a microscope, to watching colour changes on paper dipsticks. A panoply of diagnostic technologies are now available: stethoscopes, microscopy, X-rays, electrocardiograms, electroencephalograms, Doppler, echograms, ultrasound, and radioisotope, CT, MRI, and PET scans.[26]

With these tools, the doctor can link the patient's sensations to measurable changes inside her body. Our society has great confidence in signs. We believe the machines when they tell us that we are sick. We support research to invent more machines and uncover more precise signs. This state of affairs has been both celebrated and criticized.[27] The answer to the question posed at the beginning of this section explains the dilemma: sufferers from CFS do not (yet) have objective signs for their disease. Lacking a material proof of bodily change, the patient's sensations appear to be less serious, and, sometimes, less credible, as if they had been fabricated.[28] In other words, now it is possible to feel very sick and be denied the dignity of a diagnosis.

The Final Ingredient: The Observer

Signs rely on that one missing component in disease concept mixture. Did you guess what it is? The doctor, yes, or the observer, not necessarily a doctor.

During the fifteen years I have been playing the disease game, I have had the opportunity to record the responses of a wide variety of audiences: school children, undergraduates, graduates, religious groups, seniors, and voluntary organizations. All were educated and relatively well-off North Americans, and they shared many cultural values. But different groups within that context give different responses. For example, philosophy students favour words of empathy for *every* disease, not only headache. For leprosy they might write 'disfiguring'; for plague, 'sores.' Law students, on the other hand, are less often given to empathy; they cut to the chase and reach for treatments: for headache, many wrote 'ASA,' 'Tylenol,' and 'Advil'; for leprosy

Figure 1.1 Disease components that depend on the observers

Signs – objective indicators of illness

Diagnosis – what we call it

Prognosis – what we believe will happen. } Observer

Cause – what we think may cause it

Treatment – what we do to make it go away

they wrote of colonies, quarantine, prison, isolation. I should not have been surprised (but I was) when a large group of geography students managed to think of countries or continents as their first thoughts on every disease – a country for PMS? The United States, of course.

Only once did I play the word 'leprosy' and *not* encounter any responses related to the Bible. That, too, I am convinced was an observer effect. It was a group of Unitarians. I put it to them that perhaps one or two had actually thought of a biblical word first, but because of the nature of the group, they had 'cheated' and recorded a second thought. No one exactly confessed, but I saw a few guilty smiles.

In fact, if you turn back to table 1.1 and compare it with figure 1.1, nearly all the component parts of a disease concept, other than the sufferer and the illness, can be reduced to that all-important but elusive person, the observer.

The observer is the one who gets to explain the illness, to write it down, to compose the disease concept. Sometimes the observer and the sufferer are members of the same social class; sometimes a gulf of language, religion, culture, and education separates them. The presumed causes, treatments, signs, and outcomes are necessarily filtered through the observer's beliefs, which may not correspond to those of her patient. The observer pervades every component of a disease concept. Curiously

Figure 1.2 The disease (or Hippocratic) triangle

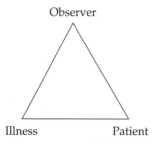

Observer

Illness   Patient

enough, the observer – that is us – is the least obvious element in our responses.

The disease game responses have changed through the short time of my experience with it, especially for the newest disease, AIDS. This too is an observer effect. In the late 1980s, words to signify homosexual men and famous individuals dominated the responses, as many participants thought first of the celebrities featured by the media: Liberace, Rock Hudson, Magic Johnson, Arthur Ashe. Now the broader scope of the disease has been assimilated to include the third world, while, curiously, blood transfusion, once a prominent cause, has vanished from the word bank of associations.

The Hippocratic Triangle

In our search to find things that diseases have in common, we have reduced the elements of disease ideas to three: the illness, the patient, and the observer. This triad is not new. In antiquity, Hippocrates was aware of the timelessness of these three components, which have come to be called the Hippocratic triangle (see figure 1.1).[29] It is a useful notion.

A disease, representing a certain person, with a certain set of symptoms, described by a certain observer, will have a 'shape' or appearance, symbolized here by the triangle, that reconciles

Figure 1.3 The disease triangle: Two observers

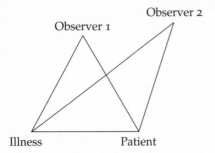

all the characteristics described above within the worldview (framework, or paradigm) of the observer.

Now imagine the same patient with the same illness, as described by a different observer, with different beliefs, values, and interests – the 'appearance' or shape of the disease might be altered (see figure 1.3). We tend to think that observers must be doctors – and indeed in our society, they hold a privileged place. But two doctors separated by two centuries will not necessarily hold the same disease concept, although their descriptions of the illness and the likely sufferers may be identical. Conversely, two people who occupy the same society but hold different worldviews – a doctor and a priest, for example – will give different accounts of a disease. The same would be true if one observer were the patient's educated employer and the other the patient's illiterate father. Again the disease might be different if the observer and the observed changed roles, and the sufferer became the observer.[30]

Accounts of diseases written by the sufferer are called 'autopathographies.' Unlike disease concepts in medical literature, which are attempts at generalizing the illness experience, autopathography is unique. We may derive useful insights from reading autopathographies, but they do not *purport* to be about more than a single person's encounter with illness. Some are

Figure 1.4 The disease triangle: Two patients

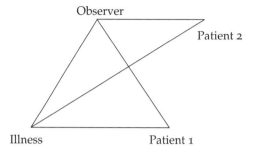

famous: for example, the writings of Hildegard of Bingen, or the late eighteenth-century surgeon John Hunter's description of what may have been his own venereal disease, or Norman Cousin's 'Anatomy of an Illness.'[31]

The triangle can be played with in a number of ways. Keeping the observer constant, but changing the patient can give some surprising results (see figure 1.4). I am reminded of the recent discovery that heart disease has been managed more laconically in women than in men.[32] A gender difference in medical approach may be scientifically justified; however, this exercise can also throw a spotlight on situations in which social biases have unintentionally, but perhaps detrimentally, crept into the disease concept. We could do the same, keeping the observer and the patient constant, and changing the symptoms.

The picture will be even more complex when observers and patients are numerous. These differences can appear even when time, place, and culture are constant. Medical anthropologist and philosopher Annemarie Mol conducted field investigations for two years in a Dutch hospital to study the varying ideas about a form of leg pain (caused by narrowed arteries and called 'intermittent claudication'). Different people – patients, internists, surgeons, pathologists, laboratory technologists – held different concepts (multiple ontologies), although they

Figure 1.5 Disease triangles based on views of people who work or are treated in the same hospital at the same time (Mol, 2002)

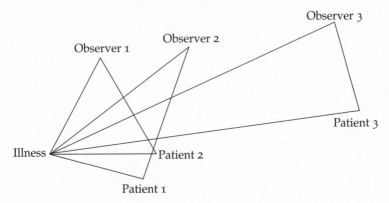

occupied the same time, place, and culture.[33] Were Mol to draw a diagram of the differing concepts of this seemingly straight-forward disease, each represented by a triangle, it might look something like figure 1.5.

The shapes of these triangles differ, symbolizing the differences in disease ideas held by patients and caregivers. In the diagram above, illness is a fixed point. But in Mol's research, even the illness – the leg pain – varied in its presence and severity. More displacements could be imagined and expressed. Problems inevitably arise when one person's pattern gets to dominate, forcing the others to conform to arrangements that do not necessarily flow from their beliefs.

Theories of Disease: What Is the Medical Model?

We have seen how individual diseases can differ, and we have been able to reduce the component characteristics of each disease to three main categories, illness, patient, and observer. But what makes a disease a disease?

If a disease concept is an explanation elaborated by an

observer of the illness experiences of one or more people, is there something that every disease must have? Can a single definition of disease work for all? Is one big theory sufficient to explain how all diseases arise and function?

Definitions of disease are almost as elusive and circular as definitions of health; they have generated an interesting philosophical literature.[34] Going back again to the disease game responses (table 1.1), let us look for a common definition of disease from the patient's perspective. Is there anything on which all sufferers of the eight conditions could agree?

They agree that disease is bad. They also hope or expect that it will go away. These simple observations constitute a theory of disease called the *organismic theory*. 'Organismic' reflects the perspective of the individual *organism* or the sufferer/patient: diseases are bad and, one hopes, discontinuous. Doctors agree. The patient consults the doctor to eliminate the problem. Disease concepts may be built from observations of collectivities, but medical practice places a high priority on the individual sufferer. The importance of the individual is apparent in the intimate manner through which the patient is interviewed and examined, and in the personalized way each person's problem is juxtaposed to all possible disease explanations (differential diagnosis). Even treatments are tailored to individual needs: age, sex, allergies, and other drugs.

The organismic theory of disease (individual, bad, and discontinuous) is the *medical model*. In the West, this theory has always held sway over medical writing. Doctors learn about diseases so that they can help solve problems in individuals. The profession of 'medicine' is named for and defined by the treatment it offers to eliminate illness, to discontinue what is bad. The intellectual business of medicine is to identify, explain, eradicate, and prevent disease. Medical epistemology, then, is nothing more, or less, than a mastery of disease concepts all built in conformation with the organismic theory.[35]

More Theories of Disease

Now let us consider two other theories that emerge from perceived causes. Sometimes the cause of an illness comes from
outside the patient – a god, a germ, a poison; sometimes it
comes from within – a gene, a behaviour, an allergy. These two
views carry certain implications. If the cause comes from outside the patient, then it exists separate from the patient and diseases will vary one from another. Which disease you have
depends on *what you have*, not on who you are. In this view, all
patients are essentially the same. This theory is called the *ontological theory*, from the Greek verb 'to be'; the cause is a 'being,'
something that exists. It conveys the advantage of absolving the
patient from blame. At the same time, it conveys the risk of
treating all sufferers in the same way, coercing (or excluding)
individuals whose symptoms do not conform to the prescribed
pattern.

On the other hand, if the cause comes from inside the patient,
then the disease cannot exist without the patient, and patients
vary more than do diseases. In this case, the disease you have
depends on *who you are*. This second theory is called the *physiological theory*, emphasizing the origin within the patient. It conveys the advantage of individualized attention. At the same
time, however, it conveys the risk of blaming patients for their
ailments.[36]

Both theories are compatible with the organismic view of disease. They have vied for dominance over the centuries. When
diseases were thought to be caused by imbalances in the four
humours of the body, the physiological view influenced the construction of all diseases. When germs were shown to be the
cause of tuberculosis in 1882, doctors anticipated that many diseases would eventually find a bacterial cause; the ontological
view then rose to predominate.[37] Many diseases, if not all, were
made to fit that conceptual framework, especially but not exclu-

sively, when the causes were unknown. The ambient scientific preoccupations of the observers shape disease construction, even when evidence may be lacking.

These two causal theories still have currency today. The ontological view operates in the diseases caused by bacteria, viruses, environmental toxins, or substance abuse. The physiological view operates in genetic, hormonal, and autoimmune diseases. Sometimes they overlap. For example, diabetes can be thought of as an insulin deficiency, arising from loss of function of the islets of Langerhans, in turn resulting from an infection-induced, autoimmunological attack on the pancreas. Similar confusion arises when we think of oncogenic viruses that 'infect' our cells by inserting themselves into our chromosomes, to be passed on as genetic material to our children and grand-children, who may then develop tumours. In these two examples, being both infectious and genetic, the mechanism is both ontological and physiological.

The ontological causal theory and the physiological causal theory overlap in another way. Since a disease takes on a life of its own when it is given a name, any disease can be spoken of as an entity, a thing, an enemy, a scourge, as if it exists – even when its cause is thought to be physiological.

One more theory will complete this picture. It stands in opposition to the medical model, just as the causal theories oppose each other. If we consider the sufferer to be not an individual but a vast collective, then we must *accept* that there will *always* be disease somewhere. This last theory holds that diseases affect populations, are always present or inevitable, and, if they are not good, they are at least tolerable. For lack of a better name, we can call it the *population theory,* or the *ecological theory,* or simply the *nonorganismic theory* of disease (see table 1.3).[38]

This last theory – the population or nonorganismic theory – has never had currency in Western medical teaching, now or in the past. Nevertheless, it informs certain religious perspectives

Table 1.3 Four theories of disease

A. Two patient-based theories	
Organismic Theory/Medical Model	*Nonorganismic/ or Population Theory*
Individuals	Populations
Bad	Good/Tolerable
Discontinuous	Continuous
B. Two cause-based theories	
Ontological theory	*Physiological theory*
Outside	Inside
Exists separate from patient	Exists only in patient
Causes vary one from another	Patients vary

on suffering; it was the basis of Malthusian philosophy or social Darwinism; and it interests health care providers who wrestle with allocation of resources, such as cut-off ages for dialysis and heart surgery, or restrictions on use of mammograms, or closure of hospitals and operating rooms.

I believe that current conflict between physicians and government resides in a fundamental conceptual disagreement: practitioners always approach illness through individuals and seek to cure each person to the best of their abilities (*organismic view*). Politicians and bureaucrats realize that eliminating all illness is impossibly utopian, and they impose limits on what can be provided, accepting that some disease is always present and that it must be tolerated (*population view*).

For similar reasons, chronic ailments, such as arthritis or neurological deficits, frustrate doctors and patients alike. Stubbornly refusing to be 'discontinuous,' incurable diseases fit poorly in the medical model. People who are dealing with a chronic problem in themselves or a family member will know exactly what I mean. Furthermore, some so-called 'sufferers' of chronic problems reject the category of disease; they refuse to label themselves as 'victims' and deny that their permanent situation is 'bad.' 'Able-ist' pressure groups raise awareness of alternative cultures and the importance of inclusion and integration; examples can be found among people who live with deafness, blindness, mental retardation, paraplegia, short stature, HIV-seropositivity, pink eyes, or missing limbs. Disease, they contend, is stigmatizing. They replace the negative 'disease' with positive words, such as 'challenge,' because they deplore what they see as the automatic implication that the condition must be 'bad' or undesirable – and, by extension, so are its sufferers. This agenda reveals once again the dominance of the organismic view of disease. Able-ists, together with religious people, anthropologists, philosophers, and some writers are prepared to find goodness, meaning, or purpose in individual suffering be it chronic or acute.[39]

The disease theories do not provide solutions to our health woes – but they offer insight. They are useful conceptual tools to help us understand disease of the present and the past. Careful reading of any text about a disease, whether it was written by a doctor, a patient, or someone else, will reveal the components of the disease concept and the theories of disease favoured by that author, thereby helping us to appreciate intellectual achievements and analyse dilemmas.

New Diseases

Diseases are sometimes said to have been 'discovered.' As we noted above, 'new diseases' will arise with changes in the elements of the disease concept, especially among causes and treatments.[40] The 'discoverer' of a disease is the observer who first distinguishes it from all other diseases. Given that a disease is an explanation, idealistic young medics might aspire to discover new diseases just as they might hope to find unknown cures. The disease may even bear his or her name: Sydenham's chorea, Hodgkin's disease, Graves' disease, Addison's disease, Bright's kidney, Cushing's syndrome – all named for doctors. Often enough, these epithets are undeserved when credit for priority goes to the wrong person, as is the case with Laennec's cirrhosis, or Down syndrome.

Indeed, the word 'discovery' is problematic. Diseases are not immutable objects lying around waiting to be unearthed like potsherds in an archaeological dig. The so-called discoverer of a disease has actually 'elaborated,' 'recognized,' 'described,' or 'invented' a new way of understanding a problem that had previously been overlooked, or forgotten, possibly because it had not been considered a problem.

Historians and sociologists like to say that diseases are 'constructed.' Beginning around 1980, a number of scholarly works were devoted to the social construction of various diseases.[41] In this view, disease ideas are 'relative' to the social position of the people who write about them. Some of these studies criticized medical practice for embedding chauvinistic judgments in its disease concepts.[42] Differences arising from race, sex, age, class, or nationality are turned into pathologies that deviate from a fallible, ethnocentric concept of 'health.' Observer bias about the 'patient' drives the disease concept, by perceiving 'illness' in differences that would be negligible were the patient and the observer to switch roles. The observer has power; the patient does not.

More recently, some historians have pulled back from the strong expression of social construction of disease. The trend was heralded by Susan Sontag, who decried the metaphors attached to cancer and tuberculosis.[43] With Sontag, social historians now recognize a biological 'reality' in the timeless manifestations of illness, even as the associated disease may change through time.[44] They also point out that patients have always held at least some power in the process of building diseases. As 'clients' or 'consumers,' they take their business elsewhere when the doctor fails to please.

Now, instead of 'disease construction,' some historians find it 'helpful' to use the more subtle term of 'framing.' For them, a disease is a biological 'reality' interpreted or embellished by culture.[45] It has become fashionable to speak of 'emerging' diseases, rather than entirely 'new' diseases.[46] According to a keyword search in Medline in early 2004, the term 'emerging disease' is emerging. It occurred once in the 1960s, 3 times between 1975 and 1979, 4 times between 1980 and 1989, 59 times between 1990 and 1999, and 87 times between January 2000 and December 2003. A medical journal entitled *Emerging Infectious Diseases* was launched in January 1995.

This steady semantic shift acknowledges the consensus-building required for an idea to achieve recognition. Die-hard critics of medical enterprise show that biological realities can be constructed, too, and remind us that we can perceive only what we are primed to seek; they point to the nature of medical epistemology as a hermeneutic product.[47]

Medicalization

A problem is 'medicalized' when it becomes the business of doctors, rather than teachers, lawyers, judges, plumbers, priests, politicians, or police. Medicalization implies the making of new diseases. For example, homosexuality was medicalized in the late nineteenth century with the collaboration and gratitude of a number of 'sufferers,' who were relieved to no longer be 'sinners' or 'criminals.'[48] It was demedicalized in 1973, by a non-unanimous vote of mostly white, mostly male, mostly heterosexual psychiatrists who agreed that homosexual orientation was no more 'sick' than it had been 'sinful' or 'criminal.'[49] An interesting research project would explore how often demedicalization has been accompanied by a collective admission either that none of the known treatments would work or that none of the patients wanted a cure.

Doctors are willing to help in a wide array of situations, but they have difficulty finding ways to intervene without first turning the problem into a disease. And to do so, they must force it to conform to the medical model, whether the fit is comfortable or not. Due to the power of the medical model, any problem that is medicalized necessarily absorbs the connotation that it is 'bad' or undesirable.

It is against this assumption that able-ists struggle in their efforts to reintegrate those identified as diseased simply because they live with disability. To date, academic law has taken a greater interest in the demedicalizing potential of able-ist thinking than has medicine.[50] In October 2002 (and again in early 2004), a Medline keyword search for 'abl(e)ist' and 'abl(e)-ist' met with zero hits. This absence is impressive, but scarcely surprising: medicine deals with disease; able-ists are intent on *de*medicalization. On the other hand, some effects are visible: the advent of cochlear implants has sparked a lively debate about deaf culture, which has left traces in the medical literature.[51] Similarly, the education literature addresses disease assumptions that are unintentionally embedded in teaching materials.[52] Able-ists, educationists, and social constructionists all warn against building diseases out of conditions that are culturally 'undesirable' or 'bad,' because these differences can emerge in, and be exaggerated by, prejudice.

In this view, medicalization is harmful. Indeed, being thought of as 'sick' can be stigmatizing. To a certain extent, we can decide that some problems should not be diseases, but cultural inclinations to perceive the situation as 'bad' are hard to shake. In his *Genesis and Development of a Scientific Fact*, Ludwik Fleck argued that the scientific efforts to perfect the Wasserman blood test for syphilis were prompted by long and deeply held convictions about disease and impure blood. With Fleck, I think that such beliefs can persist for centuries. I will give some examples in the next chapters.

Sometimes, however, there are advantages to having a disease – and not only for the child who wants to stay home from school. Creation of a disease draws attention, fosters empathy, and provides a platform for discussion, a venue for research, and a promise of cure. It can also absolve the sufferer from blame, especially, but not only, if the disease captures an ontological model for its cause. Those who grew up in the 1950s will recall that you were not to tease the fat boy: his size was not his fault, but that of his 'glands.' Groups lobby to achieve and maintain recognition of disease status. At Christmas time, during April, and always by the till of our local *dépanneur*, we are besieged by organizations appealing on behalf of sufferers from their pet condition. If you are sick, you might not have to work, and you may be entitled to benefits in terms of care, money, sympathy, and respect. Someone might even find you interesting. It sure beats going to confession, or to jail.

In our time, we are mad for medicalization. Alcoholism, smoking, infertility, prematurity, obesity, anorexia, impotence, anorgasmia, insomnia, baldness, hirsutism, sniffles, wrinkles, hot flashes, aging, anxiety, repetitive strain injury, and even shyness are problems we take to the doctor hoping for a cure. Meanwhile, newspapers inundate us with menacing reports on the advance of anthrax, Ebola, Mad Cow, West Nile virus, Lyme disease, recrudescent smallpox – and, only a few months after the reading of these lectures, SARS. And, by the way, each of these conditions has a medical historian, or two, or three, to explain its origins for us. My current favourite new disease is a condition called 'plagiocephaly,' or flat headedness of babies, which exploded across my radar screen in the summer of 2002. Toronto's Hospital for Sick Children 'has witnessed a 1,700 per cent increase in referrals to its positional plagiocephaly clinic' while the Children's Hospital of Eastern Ontario has seen a 400 per cent increase during the same period.'[53] Causes include the recent SIDS-prevention technique of placing babies on their backs and the negligence of working mothers (of course!) who park their babies in the same position for long periods of time. Treatment, available for a cost and only in some places, entails expensive little helmets, specially designed to fit and mould the infant cranium. Practitioners lament the unwillingness of the health care establishment to provide funding for the helmets. Other causes of this new 'epidemic' include the treatment, its availability, its unavailability, and the newspaper reports themselves.

In the next chapter, I will discuss the history of something that was once a disease and now, apparently, is not: the medicalization and demedicalization of romantic love. The last chapter will address a new disease: hepatitis C. In both chapters, the components of disease concepts and the four theories of disease will be used to explain the process and the problems.

To consolidate learning about the theories as they were explained in the first lecture, I assigned optional homework by inviting members of the audience to analyse four medical texts to uncover which of the disease theories had influenced the authors. The assignments were collected for marking on the second evening, and on the final evening, prizes were awarded for the best answers. For readers who would like to test their skill, the homework assignment can be found in Appendix 1.

2

Lovers: The Rise and Apparent Fall of Lovesickness

Early evening light glinting off Lake Ontario dappled the faculty club dining room in mauve and gold. The Queen's neurology department was hosting a distinguished guest speaker, and I'd been invited, because the topic, on headache, was to be historical. My dinner companion was Dr Henry Dinsdale, neurologist, former professor of medicine, and past president of the Royal College of Physicians and Surgeons of Canada. 'Did you hear?' Henry asked with his trademark enthusiasm, 'When you do PET scans of people who are in love the same parts of the brain light up as for those with OCD [obsessive-compulsive disorder]? Of course, it's old news that love is an OCD, but it's nice to have this imaging proof.'

His soft words rang like thunder in the mild May air.

Does the reduction of an emotion to a material thing – be it anatomical or chemical – allow that emotion to become a disease? This question has been asked many times before. Something measurable can easily be transformed into an 'objective' sign that can help to turn a simple trait into a disease. The process is simplified if we already harbour concerns about that trait. And, as we saw in the last chapter, disease status may afford certain advantages: it eases the burden of responsibility for those concerned – making them 'innocent victims,' 'sufferers,' or 'patients,' rather than 'bad actors,' 'criminals,' or 'sinners.' In this way, embryology and extra chromosomes came along to explain unusual behaviours and altered intellect of people who now are said to 'have' fetal alcohol syndrome, or Klinefelter's syndrome, or XYY. The discovery, measurement, and documentation of physical changes endorsed a pre-existing impulse to call these people 'sick' rather than 'bad'; they implied that 'treatment' or 'management,' rather than 'punishment' or 'incarceration,' were the appropriate reactions.

Sometimes, a newly discovered material thing is triumphantly proclaimed to be not only a sign of a disease, but also its cause and essence. Yet not all measurable deviations turn into diseases. For example, eye colour may be genetically determined, but no one chooses to see a disease in blue eyes or brown; nor does anyone fret about investigating it. Only when we *already* entertain cultural doubt about a trait or a behaviour do we construe its reduction to a material thing as a proof of its pathology. This priority of culture over biology was illustrated by the ambivalent reaction in July 1993 to the news of a 'gay gene' for homosexuality.[1] Aside from the heated controversy over the quality of the research, in which the University of Western Ontario played an important role,[2] two rival factions disputed its significance: first, those who perceive homosexual orientation as an illness, and second, those who see it as a natural variant.[3] Both groups touted the discovery as 'proof' of their opinion, as if biology trumped culture. Not only did this discovery fail to resolve the issue of whether or not homosexuality is a disease, it did even less to resolve the question of whether or not it is a sin.[4] Meanwhile, a group of ethicists perceived the possibility of harm arising from any genetic research on sexual orientation to be so great that they cautioned against engaging in such research at all.[5]

Medical epistemology is shaped just as much by society as it is by science, if not more. But it is also shaped by the medical model. To construe a material correlative as proof of a disease, we must first be prepared to imagine that the 'phenotype' – the behaviour, the symptoms, the variation – is somehow 'bad,' bad enough to hamper or endanger life, bad enough to be unwanted, bad enough to invoke the medical model or organismic theory. Then and only then do we let the material finding become a sign of disease.

So, what about love? Could it be a disease?

The answer is 'yes.' Love certainly has been considered a disease off and on since antiquity, and, until recently, more on than off. Several writers lament the paucity of words in our language for the multiple categories of love.[6] So, let me define my terms. I am not referring to fellow affection, parental fondness, deep devotion, mild enthusiasm, chipper volunteerism, or self-sacrificing patriotism. I am writing about romantic, erotic, limb-loosening, brain-befuddling, all-consuming passion. My subject is love and sex, burning desire, lust, and rest-of-your-life, self-obliterating adoration.

Lovers, like lepers, become the embodiment of their affliction. Unlike leprosy, however, the trappings of our culture show that this love is the very thing that we crave: so mighty that many religions call it God; so desirable that it must be good. How, then, could love ever have been bad enough to become a disease?

In this chapter, I will examine that question in two parts, using the concepts and theories developed in the previous chapter as tools of analysis. The first part provides an overview of the burgeoning history of lovesickness in occidental literature, including medicine, to trace its rise and apparent fall. In the second part, I will use five examples from contemporary science to demonstrate that love still qualifies as disease, notwithstanding its absence in medical school curricula. I will close with my thoughts on the reasons why. They relate to the power of the medical model (or the organismic theory) in our formulations of disease.

Audience Participation: Lovesickness among Us

On the second evening, I began by asking the audience, 'Who here has never been in love at least once? None I would guess. I won't ask for public contributions today, but for a moment of private recollection. Whether your love was requited or not, you must recall your symptoms. Please take a minute to write them down anonymously on the slips of paper provided, and I will collect them at the end of the lecture.' The results of this exercise can be seen in table 2.1.

Table 2.1 Symptoms of being in love, London, Ontario, October 2002

anorexia	irrational (2)	preoccupation with
anticipation anxiety (3)	irrational behaviour	appearance
blushing	irregular heart beat	putting other person's
breathlessness	joy	happiness above own
butterflies (3)	lack of concentration	putting person on
co-dependence	light-headedness	pedestal
conflict	little desire to eat or sleep	rapid increase in pulse
confusion	loss of appetite (2)	restlessness
constantly second-	loss of concentration	scrambled thinking
guessing	loss of rational thought	searching for person in
depression (2)	process	familiar settings
difficulty concentrating (2)	mania	self-consciousness
difficulty talking	mood swings (2)	semi-obsessive pursuit
easy laughing/crying	more responsible	sexual longing(s) (4)
elation	nausea (3)	shortness of breath
envy	nervousness	sleep disturbance
euphoria	obsessed	sleeplessness
fear	obsessive thinking,	spiritual excitement
fear of permanent	obsessive thinking,	stalker tendencies
separation	obsessive thinking ...	sweating (2)
greater understanding of	obsessive thoughts (2)	tendency to smile
people who are in love	opportunity to be emo-	foolishly
increased energy and	tional	tight chest
creativity	over-the-top exhilaration	tingling
increased interest in	over-optimism	tongue tied
romantic songs, litera-	palpitations	total 'discombobulation'
ture, etc.	perpetual preoccupation	trouble breathing
insomnia (2)	pessimism	unbreakable optimism
interest in sex manuals/	poetic skills	verbal fluency
studies	pounding heart	

My heart beats like a war drum; it beats so hard and so loud it imprisons my soul. It beats so hard and so loud I cannot possibly comprehend that she cannot hear it; that she cannot see through the bars of my plight and long for me!

These 'symptoms' have long been known as manifestations of lovesickness, together with other similar phenomena such as intrusive thoughts, rapid pulse, genital engorgement, a sense of empowerment or of weakness, trembling, impulsive behaviour, easy crying and laughing, repetitive dreams, exhilaration, desire to please, fear of rejection, jealousy, and clumsiness. When love is not mutual, the symptoms can incite misery, depression, and even death by starvation, suicide, or murder.

Love has profound physical and psychological effects. Over the centuries, these well-known effects were taken as the unchanging 'illness' component of the changing disease concept. They threatened health, interfered with normal activity, and could lead to death.

History of Lovesickness

Lovesickness has a long history. Several engaging overviews have been written, either with a broad sweep or with restrictions to period and place.[7] Some are scholarly; some entertaining; still others angrily harp on various agendas against, for example, male chauvinism,[8] heterosexism,[9] or Christian demonization of sexuality.[10] Indeed, sex looms large in these histories of lovesickness, but so does melancholy; excellent work on the subject has been written from the latter perspective.[11]

Lovesickness in Literary Antiquity

The idea of love as a disease may have arisen first as a literary metaphor – an instance of poetry affecting medicine.[12] Medical metaphors are found in ancient Egyptian love poems, from between 1300 and 1100 BC, in which the beloved is described as 'cure' and 'physician' of the disease.[13] Archaic Greek poets also resorted to medical metaphor. Lovesickness manifested in several ways: most often, it was the exquisite pain of unrequited longing. Hesiod spoke of Eros as 'fairest among the deathless gods, who unnerves the limbs and overcomes the mind and wise counsels of all the gods and all men within them.'[14] Sappho, too, described the 'limb-loosener' and his effects:

My skin became as yellow as though in boxwood dyed
My hairs fell out, and all my frame wasted to skin and bone
Was there a wizard in the town whose arts I had not tried?
A magic haunt unvisited, or cave of sibyl lone?[15]

In another fragment, she wrote,

[W]hen I look at you ... no speaking
    is left in me

no: tongue breaks and thin
fire is racing under skin
and in eyes no sight and drumming
    fills ears

and cold sweat holds me and shaking
grips me all, greener than grass
I am and dead – or almost
    I seem to me.'[16]

Love could prove fatal. A legend originating a few centuries after her death holds that Sappho threw herself from the heights of Leucadia for unrequited love, the first lover to make a suicidal leap (plate 2.1). In Euripides' play of the same name, Medea is driven mad by her lustful longing for Jason; she commits the ultimate atrocity when she murders her own children.[17] The biblical Amnon fell ill for love of his sister, Tamar; then he raped and repudiated her, for which he was murdered by his brother, Absalom (2 Sam. 13). Even when love was returned and

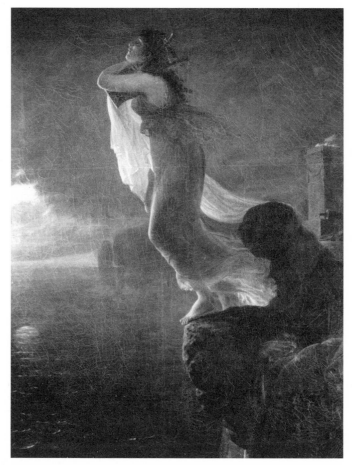

Plate 2.1 *Sappho at Leucadia* (1801) by Jean-Antoine Gros (1771–1835), Musée Baron Gérard, Bayeux, France.

sustained, it was a source of vulnerability and suffering in body and soul. In this way, Homer sang of Odysseus and Penelope's yearning for each other.[18]

Other ancient writers, including Lucian, Plutarch, Catullus, Lucretius, and Virgil, pushed the metaphor to greater lengths, but none so much as Ovid, ironic poet-laureate of the arts of love.[19] Especially in his *Remedia amoris* Ovid borrowed the by-then-well-established metaphor to satirize the nearly hopeless exercise of preventing and curing love.[20] 'Beware of solitudes,' he wrote, and 'of reading again the treasured letters.'[21] 'Drink more than your heart craves for plenty destroys passion.'[22] 'Be with someone first; find someone in whom the first bliss may spend itself; that which follows will be slow to come.'[23] Debase the object of desire, he advised, and emphasize her defects: 'say she is ugly.'[24] He offered the example of a man who 'cured' his lovesickness by contriving to watch 'while the girl performed her obscenities, and saw what even custom forbids to see.' In crafty contradiction, he continued, 'heaven forbid that I should give anyone such counsel!'[25] 'The disease has a thousand forms, I have a thousand remedies,'[26] but 'too late is the medicine prepared, when the disease has gained strength.'[27] 'A sick Podalirius, I treated myself with my own herbs, and, I confess, I was a shamefully sick physician.'[28]

In Cicero's discussion that pits the Stoics against the Peripatetics, love is a disease of the soul that can lead to disease of the body. The Stoics scorned the kind of love that is accompanied by lust, but Cicero, possibly relying on Aristotle, doubted that there was any other kind: 'if in the actual world there is an instance of love free from disquietude from longing from anxiety from sighing, then so be it!' He defined love as an intense belief that regards a thing as desirable; for a cure, he offered Ovid's lame, therapeutic strategy of trying to transform the coveted object into one of contempt.[29]

Ancient literary sources are divided about the prospect of treatment for the metaphorical ailment. Theophrastus held that 'Love is the excess of some irrational desire which is quickly acquired and slowly got rid of'; it is 'the passion of an idle mind.'[30] With blithe disregard for tenacious relationships, some recommended the simple, mechanical cure of sexual congress with the loved one: painful desire, once satisfied, would wane. This remedy occurs frequently over the centuries. Plutarch (ca 45–125) and several others tell the tale of Antiochus, son of Seleucus, the King of Assyria. The young man is sick with secret love for his father's beautiful wife (or concubine) Stratonice. The worried father consults the famous Alexandrian physician Erasistratus, who quickly 'diagnoses' the problem and uses deception to solve it. First, the doctor asks the anxious parent if he would refuse anything in order to restore his son to health. Having extracted the anticipated reply, the doctor then demonstrates that the lad's cure must be union with the woman, and the father is honour-bound by the doctor's ruse to marry his son to his wife.[31] This story was repeated so often that one nineteenth-century writer observed that it was known to 'everyone.'[32]

Other authors, including Sappho and Ovid, pretended that a cure was impossible, if not undesirable. The first-century Latin poet Propertius seems to have equated his literary lovesickness with madness; he followed the medical cures for insanity as described by his contemporary, Celsus,[33] in expressing the arduous task of curing love:

> Medicine's for pain but of pain only love loves no artful alleviation … if a man can remove this grievous love from my heart, that same man can hand an apple to Tantalus and … unloose Prometheus from his cliff and beat off the vultures feeding on his belly.[34]

In short, the cure for literary lovesickness demands prowess greater than that of the gods. Now, how could any self-respecting physician resist such a challenge? Doctors eventually got involved, but they did so slowly. In medical antiquity, as opposed to literary antiquity, love was not yet a full-blown disease. Rather it was an imitator of disease, while its *excess* – or more precisely, excess sex – might be harmful.

Lovesickness in Ancient Medical Sources

In the fifth century BC, the Hippocratic author warned that disease could arise through abuse of love's pleasures, either from overuse ('venery') or from underuse, as in the case of young virgins who failed to marry; moderation was key.[35] A later legend, described in the Hippocratic biography of Soranus of Ephesus (first or second century AD), had the Father of Medicine distinguishing lovesickness from consumption in one Perdiccas, prince of Macedonia; however, here again, love is not a disease per se, and the tale is thought to have been borrowed from the legend about Erasistratus (described above).[36]

In the second century AD, Galen wrote of love more frequently than had his medical predecessors. He agreed with Hippocrates about the physiological importance of moderation in passionate emotions and sexual activity,[37] also claiming that too little indulgence was just as dangerous as too much.[38] On lovesickness, however, his purpose was to distinguish it from 'real' diseases, such as melancholy, which he conceived of as a physical excess of black bile. In Galen's view, the pulse was altered by strong emotion and could be used to identify love in opposition to disease. It was by feeling a pulse that Erisistratus had made his impressive diagnosis of the son's love for his father's wife. In the same way, Galen recognized love in a Roman lady whom other physicians had thought of as sick: her pulse faltered when the dancer Pylades was mentioned in conversation.[39]

In the first century AD, Aretaeus the Cappadocian told a similar story of a youth thought to be suffering from intractable melancholy: 'when the physicians could bring him no relief, love cured him.' Aretaeus decided that the ailment had been wrongly diagnosed by unsophisticated observers as a real disease. He wrote:

> But I think he was originally in love, and that he was dejected and spiritless from being unsuccessful with the girl, and appeared to

the common people to be melancholic. He then did not know that it was love; but when he imparted the love to the girl, he ceased from his dejection, and dispelled his passion and sorrow; and with joy he awoke from his lowness of spirits, and he became restored to understanding, love being his physician.[40]

Clearly Aretaeus, like Galen, distinguished melancholy from love. As the young man was not suffering from true melancholy, 'success' with the girl was a 'cure' for what merely appeared to be disease.[41] Here the physician borrowed the metaphor of the poets.

Scientific writers, including Aristotle, had been interested in emotions, including love, and some authors debated the anatomical location of these powerful feelings as the brain or the heart.[42] But emotions were not diseases, even if they mimicked them; emotions were epiphenomena of existence.[43] Love might perhaps be an antecedent cause of mania, or of melancholy, or of a melancholy-like state; however, that too was under dispute. Until the second century AD then, love was a disease in poetry, song, and philosophy, but apparently not in medicine.

Things began to change by the fourth century AD, when the well-respected pagan physician Oribasius of Pergamum (326–403) accepted the task of curing lovesickness. Like other diseases of the time, his lovesickness featured insomnia and sadness, but it could be distinguished by the additional signs of hollow, dry eyes and fluttering eyelids. In his chapter 'On Lovers,' Oribasius recommended wine, baths, passive movement, and the diversions of music and theatre, 'for the passion of those who are incessantly preoccupied by their love is difficult to uproot.'[44] Rather than seeing lovesickness as a metaphor and separating love as a nondisease from 'real' diseases, Oribasius wrote about unrequited, passionate love as a distinct entity, a disease project *sui generis*, for physicians to diagnose and treat. He also came up with an additional method for distracting intransigent lovers bent on wallowing in their misery: they must be 'frightened.'[45] Oribasius's words were repeated and amplified some three centuries later, by Paulus Aegineta, in his chapter 'On Lovesick Persons.' Paulus rejected the opinion of Galen and others that special signs were to be found in the pulse.[46] He agreed that lovers 'must be attacked with fear'[47] – a strategy, it seems, much like saying 'Boo!' to a person with hiccups.

The familiar similarities between love and melancholy seem to have led 'some physicians' to recommend love as a cure for mania, which was seen as the opposite of melancholy. But the fifth-century Latin physician Caelius Aurelianus disputed the idea of love as a cure for insanity, notably mania. His reasons were relentlessly logical:

> Some physicians hold that love is a proper remedy for insanity on the ground that it frees the patient's mind from the agitation caused by madness and thus purifies it ... they are not aware of the obvious truth that in many cases love is the very cause of the madness. Nor should we disdain the vices of those who had actually called love a form of insanity because of the similarity of the symptoms which the victims show. And surely it is absurd and wrong to recommend of all remedies for the disease the very thing that you are trying to treat, not to mention the fact that it is impossible to get an insane person to fall in love, for, since he is bereft of reason, he cannot properly appreciate beauty.[48]

With these words, Caelius made it clear that love was not only a full-blown disease, but a *cause* of disease.

Another influential writer of antiquity was more philosophical than he was poetic or medical: Saul of Tarsus, or Saint Paul. Passages on love from his first epistle to the Corinthians (13.1–13) are often cited, most famously in the recent past by British Prime Minister Tony Blair at the funeral of Diana Princess of Wales. Paul sundered two components of erotic love, separating the emotion (which was worthy) from carnality (which was not). When the sexual urge was overwhelming, Paul grudgingly acknowledged that it was 'Better to marry than to burn' (1 Cor. 7.9). Of small consequence, perhaps, at the time of writing, this artificial duality between lust and love came to pervade and preoccupy Christian thought, creating moral dilemmas for lovers who were interested in procreation, for those who were not, and for doctors who tried to care for them all.[49]

Medieval Lovesickness

Some scholars contend that Western medicine learned to think of love as a disease from tenth-century Persian doctors. Both al-Razi (Abu-Bakr Mohammed Ibn Zakaria Al-Razi, or Rhazes, 865?–965?) and Ibn Sina (or Avicenna, 980–1037) wrote on lovesickness. For them, it was a form of insanity stemming from erotic desire, the cure for which was sexual intercourse. They gave the malady special new names: for Rhazes it was 'coturub';[50] for Ibn Sina, 'illisci.'[51] Unlike his contemporaries and predecessors, however, Ibn Sina wrote favourably about the equal importance of women's pleasure for conception. Other treatises on lovesickness were written by the Islamic physicians Ali b. Muhammad al-Dailami, thought to be an older contemporary of Ibn Sina,[52] and by Ibn al Jazzar; the latter's work was translated into Latin at least twice in the eleventh century.[53]

These Persian teachings are said to have mollified medical opinion on sexual practices as natural and effective cures at a time when Christian influences and rules demanded restraint.[54] But love had long been a well-developed disease concept in the minds of poets and philosophers, and the lovesickness of these Islamic writers is similar to that of the earlier Oribasius and Paulus. Their writings certainly codified the older idea; however, it is difficult to claim that lovesickness originated in the Middle East, although it may have been medicalized there as an isolated 'discovery,' independent of Mediterranean influence. Sustaining my argument about the pervasive, cultural willingness to pathologize love, disease imagery is also found in the work of early Islamic poets[55] and in the folk wisdom of Hindu, Japanese, Chinese, and Irish cultures.[56]

The most important medical writer for the medieval history of lovesickness was Constantine the African (d. 1087). A monk at Montecassino, Constantine began the long work of translating ancient, medical wisdom back into Greek and Latin from the Middle Eastern languages in which it had resided for several centuries.[57] In Constantine's *Viaticum*, love was a full-blown disease, characterized by hollow eyes, great longing, and intense sexual desire; it was akin to melancholy, both in its manifestations and its cause as humoral imbalance.[58] If untreated, the lover could fall into an intractable depression. The cure was evacuation of excess humours by the usual methods, including bleeding, baths, and sexual intercourse. Curious to us, perhaps, the sexual treatments seemed to pose no ethical dilemma for the religious scribes.[59] Other therapies could help too: 'temperate and fragrant wine, listening to music, conversing with dearest friends, recitation of poetry, looking at bright, sweet smelling, fruitful gardens, clear running water' and amusements 'with good-looking women or men.' Constantine may have taken his ideas from a now-missing treatise on melancholy by Rufus of Ephesus (second century AD), which he cited.[60]

Following Constantine, who used the word 'eros,' and his student, Johannes Afflacius, who used the word 'heros,' lovesickness acquired yet another name, which was rendered as 'amore heroico' by the thirteenth-century physician Arnaldus of Villanova (d. 1311). Others called it 'hereos.' Scholars have invested much ink in trying to unravel the origin and meaning of this name, which mysteriously invokes both the sensually erotic and the militaristically heroic.[61]

Arnaldus's short Latin treatise 'De amore heroico' is known

to exist in only four manuscripts; a critical edition was published in 1985 by the distinguished medievalist Michael McVaugh.[62] For Arnaldus, lovesickness was defined as the 'joyous perception of a desirable object,' and it featured the by-now-familiar symptoms of anorexia, insomnia, and melancholy. Arnaldus emphasized the physiological consequences, which included overheating of the spirits in the heart, the brain, and the entire body. Although the problem was anchored in the body, the process corresponded to other contemporary writings about what we would now call 'mental illness': at the time, these problems were conceived as physical, not psychic, disorders.[63]

The extent of Arnaldus's influence is difficult to determine because the metaphorical and medical associations of love and disease had already been intertwined for more than 1500 years. Nevertheless, his works appear to have been widely known. Variations on the word 'hereos' turn up in many lay writings, and Arnaldus is cited by literary scholars of medieval England, France, Germany, Italy, and Spain.[64] Thus, Boccaccio, Andreas Cappellanus, Cavalcanti, Chaucer, Dante, Petrarch, Rojas, Thomas, and the unknown author of the *Carmina Burana* have all been exposed as secret readers of contemporary medicine, whether or not they knew their Ovid.[65] Some scholars are enthusiastic about the evident links to medicine and urge their literary colleagues to turn to contemporary medical prose for insight into the poetry and philosophy of their periods.[66] Far be it from me to discourage the reading of medical history, but here surely is an example of misattribution: when it comes to the disease of love, the poets were there long before the doctors.

Courtly love presents a special debate in current scholarship.[67] This idealistic, self-sacrificing, but not-so-sexy version of love is thought to have originated with Gaston of Paris and the twelfth-century erudite cleric Andreas Capellanus, who referred to love as a sad malady. Scholars are divided: either courtly love was a pervasive social ideal or it was simply a satirical device.[68] Capellanus offers a pretty argument between a man and a woman on whether or not there can be love and jealousy in marriage. It is resolved by the Countess of Champagne, in a letter supposedly dated 1 May 1174 in which she said 'no' – neither love nor jealousy can exist in marriage because the spouses already have physical possession of each other.[69] To counter this apparent endorsement of open marriage, Capellanus's third book lays out twelve grim consequences of extramarital love.[70] In condemning adultery, he also condemns women who inspire it, as if they are the cause of the disease.[71] Recent criticism contends that Andreas Capellanus was only joking but that he lacked the fire of Ovid to make it plain.[72]

Early Modern Lovesickness

In the medical Renaissance, many diseases were given fuller descriptions. A rising trend emphasized detailed observations of symptoms and would eventually culminate in a self-conscious enterprise called 'nosology' (see chapter 1).[73] Doctors were looking for more symptoms and treatments for all diseases. Love was no exception. Without abandoning the older formulations, doctors imposed on lovesickness the trappings of early modern science and social values.

Early in the sixteenth century, a frightening new condition riveted attention on the dangers of physical love: syphilis. In his treatise on the 'French disease,' Fracastoro warned his readers to 'fly from desire and the soft embraces of love, for nothing is more harmful.'[74] Although his purpose may have been to promote mercury as treatment and he included several potential causes, his words indicate that he knew that sex could spread this disease. Let me be clear: as a disease, syphilis was always separate from lovesickness. Nevertheless, the recognition of syphilis as a mortal peril enhanced medical interest in the problem of affectionate attraction. Syphilis also served to promote more stringent attitudes toward sex and frivolity, a direction that the Church had officially been urging for centuries, but one that clerical scribes and the medics who treated the lovelorn had previously been able to ignore.

The most impressive medical work on lovesickness from this period was the lengthy treatise of Jacques Ferrand (b. 1575). He gave the disease yet another name: 'erotomania.'[75] Donald Beecher of the University of Ottawa published a translation in 1990. Using a brilliant comparison between two editions of 1610 and 1623, Beecher showed how the long-standing medical leniency toward sex as therapy may have come into conflict with the authorities who were directing the Inquisition. For his second edition, Ferrand retracted some of the tried-and-true wisdom of his predecessors, including the useful technique of coitus with a bawd.[76] In all other respects, Ferrand's erotomania is the familiar disease of body and soul that had been recognized for centuries by doctors and poets alike.

Other works from the medical Renaissance featured citations from the ancients. Daniel Sennert (1572–1637) of Germany wrote of 'amore insano' as a form of melancholy. Citing a host of medical authors and poets both ancient and modern, including Ovid, Ibn Sina, and Ferrand, Sennert claimed that this lovesickness was easy to cure in its initial stages. If left untreated, however, insane love could degenerate into mania, marasmus, and death by suicide.[77] André Du Laurens (1558–1609) of Montpellier also viewed love as both a type and a cause of melancholy with dangerous side effects. Relying on Plutarch's old story of Erasistratus and the son of Seleucus, he described two cures: 'enjoyment of the object of love,' or the 'artifice and industry of an excellent physician.' To dispel the myth that drinking blood of the beloved was an effective remedy, Du Laurens retold the story of Faustina. Though she was married to Marcus Aurelius, Faustina fell for a gladiator. The jealous emperor had the man killed and slipped his wife a drink spiked with her lover's blood. She was cured of her passion, but from the next union with her husband sprang the demonic emperor Antonius Commodius, whose notorious cruelty, on this reading, turns out to have been a colossal, iatrogenic disaster.[78] Were these passages written in earnest? As practitioners, how often did the authors actually diagnose and treat lovesickness? Or, were these chapters elegant diversions intended to display fashionable erudition and to alleviate the tedium of ponderous medical prose?

Contemporary Renaissance values crept into formulations of love as a disease. In a rising tide of misogyny, women, who had long been thought of as the object and even cure of the obsession, now became its evil yet irresistible cause.[79] Lucas Cranach's exquisite Venus with her honey-sweet, bee-stung Cupid reflects this attitude (plate 2.2).

In keeping with the pervasive medical preoccupation of the nosologists for disease classifications, special distinctions were splintered off to become new diseases, including 'nymphomania,' 'narcissism,' and 'tarantism.'[80] Contracting one of these diseases allowed for sexual expression that might otherwise be socially proscribed. The disease chlorosis, or the green sickness of virgins, seems to have been yet another variant of lovesickness, as described in the 1544 treatise of Johannes Lange (1485–1565). It too satisfied social and political functions. Now equated with both anorexia nervosa and with iron deficiency anemia, the clinical manifestations of this disease were similar to those of lovesickness, and the cure – marriage as soon as possible – was the unmistakable legacy of both Hippocrates and Ovid.[81]

Meanwhile, the metaphor of love as disease persisted in the arts. Robert Burton (1577–1640), among others, resorted to it in his *Anatomy of Melancholy*, the first of its many editions appearing in 1621.[82] Lovesickness also spawned a genre of painting, typified by the work of Jan Steen and other seventeenth-century

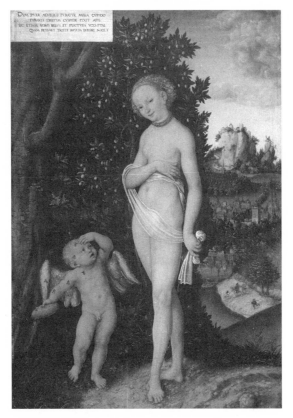

Plate 2.2 *Venus and Cupid with Honeybees* (1530) by Lucas Cranach, Statens Museum for Kunst, Copenhagen, Denmark.

Dutch painters, who featured encounters between women ailing from heartache and their physicians (plates 2.3 and 2.4).[83] Similarly, music was written to soothe the pains of the lovelorn.[84] Sex manuals aimed at the literate public appeared in multiple editions, perhaps because the unhealthy implications of a frustrated love life had captured and alarmed a wide audience.[85]

AMORVM.

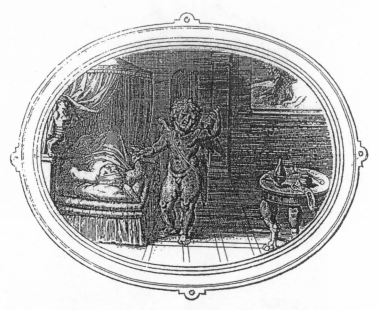

Plate 2.3 'One Love Cures Another,' by Otto van Veen, Amorum Emblemata, *Amans Amanti Medicus*, 1608.

Writers of the eighteenth century, including Voltaire, Swift, and Goethe, equated the sickness arising from love with venereal disease, or with the draconian side effects of its mercurial treatments – if they used the disease metaphor at all.[86]

Perhaps the poets were bored with the much-used medical metaphor of love as a disease. After many centuries of popularity, it may have seemed a quaint and tired cliché for expressing the emotional state of overwrought youth. Writers turned to other literary devices to express their awe of love, and they left its medicalization to the doctors. Imbued with the nosological passion for classification, the latter found wonderful new ways

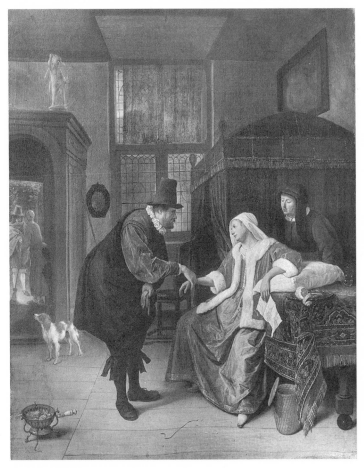

Plate 2.4 *The Lovesick Woman* (ca 1660) by Jan Steen, Bayerische Staats-gemaldesammlungen.

to further multiply and subdivide the manifestations of the malady. In the eighteenth century, lovesickness and its variations blossomed into a distinct component of medical school curricula all across Europe.

Erotomania Goes Modern and Seems to Disappear

In 1724, eighteen-year-old François Boissier des Sauvages (1706–67) successfully defended his medical thesis on the disease of love, refuting the claim, cited from Ovid, that lovesickness was incurable.[87] Sauvages went on to write a much larger and important treatise to classify all diseases. In his later works, he retained lovesickness as 'amorous melancholy,' a type of 'delirium,' within the class of 'vesanias' (mental disorders). He distinguished it from 'nymphomania' and 'satyriasis,' which were also diseases of the mind without 'delirium.'[88]

Sauvages's contemporaries and followers also kept a disease category for love. Jerome David Gaub (1705–80), a German who taught at Leiden, classified it as a disease of lifestyle and warned that excess of love, either as sex or as emotion, could provoke serious physical disease.[89] William Cullen (1712–90) of Edinburgh and several other eighteenth-century authors, including Carolus Linnaeus (1707–78), continued to classify erotomania as a form of melancholy.[90]

From the sixteenth to the nineteenth centuries, while the nosologist-clinicians sorted diseases by symptoms, medical scientists were preoccupied with the anatomical localization of symptoms. Anticipating this preoccupation and confirming yet again his scientific fluency, Shakespeare wrote, 'Tell me where is fancy bred / Or in the heart or in the head?'[91] As the causes and seats of diseases were situated in the organs, the tradition of identifying diseases by their symptoms was challenged. But mental disorders did not easily mesh with this new anatomical agenda. So began a huge debate, which is still unresolved: whether or not mental diseases could be localized in the body. If love was a neurosis, its locus and treatment were obscure. Failing to find a place in these rising organic preoccupations, lovesickness was left to the psychiatrists.

For example, the psychiatrist Jean-Étienne-Dominique

Esquirol (1772–1840) included erotomania as a type of 'mono-mania' or irrational fixation on a single object, much like obsession today. Committed to integrating anatomy with psychiatry, Esquirol situated his erotomania in an as-yet-unknown lesion of the brain, as opposed to 'nymphomania' and 'satyriasis,' which he placed in the genitals.[92]

But make no mistake: be it psychic or physical, love could still be dangerous. Napoleon's personal physician, the internist Jean-Nicolas Corvisart (1755–1821), described the physical impact of erotic love upon the heart: 'A lover dies at the very moment the flame of his passion was to be satisfied ... apparently thunderstruck with a paroxysm of passion.'[93] Stendhal's 1822 novel *De l'amour* was based on an extended and almost antiquated metaphor of love as a disease. Emerging from a bitter personal experience, he likened love to a malignant fever that weakened the brain.[94]

Soon lovesickness was further subdivided into yet more categories, such as masturbation, homosexuality, and pedophilia. Most forms of lovesickness were sexual. Previously they had been sins; now they were elaborations of 'perversities' or deviations from the hegemony of 'natural' heterosexual attraction.[95] At this point, lovesickness begins its apparent decline.

The Turning Point

No longer restricted to unrequited desire, the diseases (now plural) of love were invented and characterized as 'unnatural' desires, which doctors were invited to diagnose and treat.[96] Nineteenth-century writers of fiction became interested in the new diseases of sexual perversity, just as their predecessors had been interested in lovesickness.[97] Popular images of lovesick women trivialized, dramatized, and infantilized the emotion and have been described as yet another tool of misogynist social control (plate 2.5).[98]

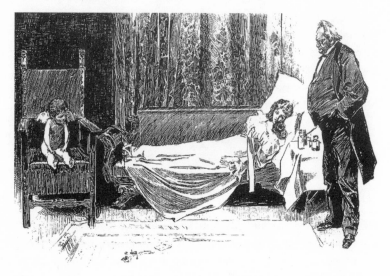

Plate 2.5 The lovesick Gibson girl: 'When Doctors Disagree' from *The Gibson Girl and Her America*, ed. Edmund Gillon, Jr. (Dover 1969), 32.

Doctors do not 'invent' diseases in a vacuum. They can do little, epistemologically speaking, without a willing market. Using the example of homosexuality in the late nineteenth century, Bert Hansen has shown how patients' requests for help charted this course as much as, if not more than, their doctors' proclivity to 'take over' new territory.[99] Similarly, Judith Leavitt draws attention to the role of expectant mothers in the medicalization of birth.[100] In both situations, medicine followed society; having done so, it did what it had always done and turned to science for justification.

The genitals were, if anything, a more frequent site of disease than they are now. Following this shift to organ-based definitions of disease, surgical cures were conceptually tempting. As soon as the mid-nineteenth-century discoveries of anesthesia and antisepsis made operations relatively safe, they became fashionable. Ovariotomy was used to treat a host of complaints in women, simply, it seems, because the sufferers were female.[101] However, the diseases that were localized to the genitals were no longer seen to be problems of love. If they were pathologized at all, love and other emotions stubbornly remained in the old-fashioned classification system based on symptoms that applied to mental illness.[102]

Reformers of the late nineteenth and early twentieth centuries, like George Drysdale, Marie Stopes, Havelock Ellis, Margaret Sanger, and H.G. Wells, sought to re-legitimize aspects of sexuality and launched a crusade to promote birth control and social tolerance.[103] But, with the exception of Wells, they travelled a delicate course: heterosexual love within marriage was good; all else was bad, albeit bad enough for disease, not for sin.

And then came Sigmund Freud. I will not attempt to rehearse the content or impact of his vast work on emotions and sexuality. Suffice it to say that he *de*-pathologized so much of what had once been 'sick,' especially as it pertained to heterosexual men. In his wake, sociologists, physiologists, and psychologists began to study erotic relationships with the anodyne goal of description and demystification. The names of Alfred C. Kinsey, William Masters and Virginia Johnson, Erich Fromm, and Shere Hite spring to mind.[104] But perhaps one of the most intriguing if less appreciated works of this nature is that of Montreal journalist Pierre Léger, who in the 1960s published the results of his survey of 146 *québécoises* under the spellbinding title *La canadienne française et l'amour, ou L'homme démystifié*. The paperback puffed itself somewhat disingenuously as bedside reading (*'livre de chevet'*) with the recommendation that 'chacun devrait le lire pour mieux se comprendre et accepter l'autre.'[105]

In the wake of the birth-control pill, sex came right out of the closet and one by one the diseases of physical love were gradually defrocked. The manual *The Joy of Sex*, featuring clean line drawings of a suburban couple enjoying congress in various postures, made sexual resourcefulness resemble culinary skill, as something every 1960s homemaker should be able to provide, in between voting, working full-time, driving the kids to school, pressing shirts, and delivering keynote lectures – an elusive project almost as quixotic as being Twiggy-thin![106] And soon appeared the books that begin 'get a mirror, go in the bathroom, and close the door.'

Sex was considered healthy and fun – everyone ought to have it – and some doubted that messy, emotional love needed to be involved at all. Homosexuality was formally removed from the *Diagnostic and Statistical Manual (DSM)* in 1973, and sex as therapy made a comeback from the Middle Ages in 1988, when 'Sex Counselling' became a Medical Subject Heading for Medline. Even masturbation was given a nudge in the direction of medical sanction by U.S. Surgeon General Jocelyn Elders in December 1994, not without dramatic repercussions that included her forced resignation.[107]

It is difficult to overemphasize the extent to which sex talk has become mainstream. Upon my return from sabbatical in August 2002, I was invited by e-mail to the University women's centre to attend a seminar on 'women's sexuality, orgasm and sex toys.' The message urged female members of the Queen's community to 'Discover creative ways to keep the spark in your sex life. Add new twists to your routine. Learn about orgasm and that ever elusive G-spot. Explore playfulness and sex toys.'[108] At first, I thought that our university's anti-spamming device had sprung another leak until I realized that this message hailed from within. Of course, only some sexual behaviours have moved into the realm of normal: for example, degrading and sadomasochistic practices occupy a grey area, while pedophilia, necrophilia, and sexual violence, including rape, are considered so offensive that they remain crimes, even if they may also be manifestations of disease.[109]

Some scientists, far from seeking to cure romantic love, are now inclined to tout its benefits for individual and species survival. They postulate ecological explanations for why we might experience 'falling in love.' Physicians and patients alike had long thought that a happy state of mind was beneficial for health. By the early 1960s, Jonas Salk speculated that the similarities between reticulo-endothelial cells and nervous tissue might imply links between mental state and immunity.[110] Then an exciting discovery, announced in 1973, uncovered evidence of mind–body links in the form of opiate receptors and endorphins.[111] These internally generated, feel-good hormones dope us up when we are happy, helping us to resist infection and malignancy. The location of endorphin receptors in the brain and gut explained many gastrointestinal symptoms of nervousness, fear, and other excitement.[112] Studies of endorphins, entailing avoidable and unavoidable shocks to the feet of animals, suggested that misery hampers immunity and enhances tumour growth.[113]

Candace Pert, one of the American discoverers of opiate receptors, has become a scientific poster-girl for mind–body medicine: she claims that the things that raise our neuropeptides – positive emotions, good workouts, good food, good sex, and good loving – are the key to good health.[114] Along similar lines, a group working in Pisa, Italy, demonstrated that the blood platelets of lovers are less sticky than average, which might mean fewer thrombosis-causing clots on those love-induced, hormonal occasions – such as pregnancy – that normally raise the risk.[115] A Medline search on the keywords 'broken heart' will turn up articles on therapeutic interventions from psychiatry to cardiac surgery.

By now you ought to be convinced of two things: first, love was once a well-established, card-carrying disease; and second, sometime in the twentieth century, its disease status appeared to vanish. If anything, love now seems to be good for us.

Is Love Still a Disease?

So, love is no longer a disease, right? Wrong! I believe it still carries disease overtones in the medical and cultural psyche, for many of the same reasons it was always thought of as 'bad.' Fine examples continue to emerge in literature, music, and art. In Brian Moore's novel *The Doctor's Wife*, the protagonist falls in love with a younger man. Her husband and her brother, both doctors, can understand only by imagining that she must be sick.[116] Joan Connor's brilliant short story 'How to Stop Loving Someone: A Twelve-Step Programme' satirizes lovesickness as well as the popular proclivity to medicalize.[117] In May 2000, an epidemic computer virus rapidly spread around the world, costing billions of dollars and causing massive disruption to the hapless victims who 'fell for' it by opening the wicked attachment that infected their computers and destroyed their electronic and financial savings. How much less would the damage have been had the seductive virus not said 'I love you'?[118] And on Valentine's Day 2002, the third most popular love song in France (after Edith Piaf's 'Hymne d'amour' [in English 'If you love me'] and Jacques Brel's 'Ne me quitte pas'), was Michel Sardou's rendition of the 1973 song 'La maladie d'amour.' Ask any Frenchman about lovesickness and he will burst into song.

For the remainder of this chapter, however, I will stick to the pathology of love within medical science, drawing my evidence from five examples in three broad domains of research: psychiatry, neuroscience, and addiction. A reminder – the focus is not sexuality alone, although that is part of it. The focus is still erotic, limb-loosening, falling-in-love-with-love, romantic love.

Psychiatry: Examples 1, 2, and 3

It may come as a surprise, but erotomania is still a bona fide diagnosis in psychiatry. Homosexuality may have been removed from the *DSM-IIIR* nearly thirty years ago, but erotomania persists even into the current fourth edition of 1994. It is classified as a type of 'delusional disorder' in which the afflicted, most often a female, is in love with a 'person usually of a higher status' – such as a movie star, musician, or sports hero.[119] She may also hold the inappropriate belief that her feelings are reciprocated. The *DSM* recognizes that patients may run into difficulty with the law as the object of their affection seeks protection from unwanted overtures, harassment, and stalking. An example, given in the *DSM* casebook, is of a fifty-five-year-old hospital-cafeteria worker who was convinced that a certain doctor was in love with her. She was treated successfully with an anti-psychotic drug and later an antidepressant.[120] This variant of lovesickness was first described in the early nineteenth century by J.E.D. Esquirol and later by Richard von Krafft-Ebing (1840–1902). Eventually, it came to be known as known as De Clérambault's syndrome, following the description of '*psychose passionelle*' by Gaétan G. de Clérambault (1872–1934), which was published posthumously in 1942. In the earlier version, special emphasis was placed on the unwarranted belief that the adored – often an older, richer man – was also in love with the patient and that he had instigated the relationship.[121] In the recent *DSM* versions, the embedded narcissism is toned down.

I could rest my case here, but the pathology of love affects many more than a handful of cranks. The second example also stems from psychiatry. Remember transference? It is a psychological mechanism discovered by Freud that the analysand could fall in love with her analyst. And counter-transference? This occurs when the feelings run in the opposite direction. After Marilou McPhedran's 1991 task force on sexual abuse of patients and the tighter rules governing physician–patient relationships in Ontario, counter-transference was partially demedicalized and newly 'criminalized' to become the basis of crime.[122] But it has also been remedicalized as a 'disease' and a subject of research. Recent articles describe treatment for the 'impaired therapist' and the sinister-sounding condition of 'malignant eroticized countertransference.'[123] I wish to neither dispute nor diminish the harm that could stem from doctors acting on those feelings, but I think it is fair to say that transference/counter-transference represent yet more neologisms and subdivisions in the convoluted history of lovesickness. These doctors are in love. At least they *think* they are in love, and who else would be a better judge? Being socially unacceptable – i.e., bad – their love can be medicalized on the organismic theory of disease.

Psychiatric epidemiology of the last decade offers a third manifestation of love as a disease, or at least as a source of harm and even death by suicide or murder. A famous case of jealous rage is that of Scarsdale diet author Herman Tarnower, who was murdered by his lover, schoolteacher Jean Harris, in March 1980.[124] Several studies, including one based on Quebec coroners' cases, have shown that 'amorous jealousy' is a cause of half the spousal murders committed by women and 90 per cent of those family tragedies of murder-suicide committed by men.[125] Love, then, can led to premature death.

We can try to get around the medicalizing implications of these psychiatric examples by qualifying all the different categories – the erotomanic, the transferant, the suicidal, and the murderous – by saying 'That's jealousy, anger, depression. That's not *real* love!' Indeed, we hope it is not love. But would the subjects agree? I think not. And, actions aside, who are we to redefine someone else's emotion?

Neuroscience: Example 4

Neuroscience is the specialty of Henry Dinsdale, my dinner companion at the beginning of this chapter. Recall he reported that lovers' brains 'light up' like those of people with obsessive-compulsive disorder (OCD).

In the mid-1970s, soon after the discovery of opiate receptors and endorphins, researchers began to study the brain location of sophisticated mental processes that had previously eluded detection: emotions, memories, moods, and dreams. Magnetic resonance imaging (MRI) and positron emission tomography (or PET scan) are remarkable devices for displaying brain function as well as structure. Earlier imaging methods, such as X-rays and computerized tomography (CT scan) were fairly static; they showed brain structure and blood flow, but they were silent on other dynamic processes. Now it is possible to trace the path, distribution, and metabolism of specific chemicals, locating them in both time and space within the brain. PET scanning is active; its precursors were more passive.

Because PET scans are expensive, most studies use only a small number of subjects and their design wrestles to avoid cultural assumptions. For example, in a project to study the brain location of memory for pleasant and aversive stimuli, ten healthy male volunteers were given PET scans while being shown pleasant, unpleasant, and neutral pictures on two occasions, four weeks apart. What were the pictures? Those classified as 'aversive' were of 'diseased bodies, frightening animals, and lethal violence'; neutral pictures were of 'chess players, plants, and household scenes'; and pleasant pictures included 'appealing animals, appetizing food, and sexually arousing scenes.'[126] A study of a handful of men, designed and conducted by men, and published in a distinguished journal in 1999.

In the interests of gender equality, let us focus on a different PET scan study done on female subjects in 1997. To localize the feelings of happiness, sadness, and disgust, twelve right-handed women were subjected to PET scanning while being shown two-minute-long silent film clips. The all-male authors restricted the study to women, for 'homogeneity,' they wrote, and to 'enhance emotional response.' In this case, 'disgust' was to be provoked by a scene of a rat crawling on a sleeping man;

'sadness,' by the death of a friend; and 'happiness,' by joyous reconciliation – presumably her guy coming home from the hot sexual fantasy he had enjoyed in the last experiment.[127] The subjectivity of science roars loudly. These authors sagely tell us that the concept of basic emotions originated with Darwin in 1872. Darwin? What about Aristotle? or Theophrastus?

PET scanning becomes even more intriguing when it is applied to treatment of mental disorders. Recently, investigators have identified the parts of the brain involved with various anxiety 'disorders' such as post-traumatic stress disorder, panic disorders, and obsessive-compulsive disorder (OCD).[128] By 'tagging' or labelling the drugs used to treat these conditions, researchers can study whether or not they concentrate in the parts of the brain implicated in the problem. For example, a group working on the brain location of OCD used PET scanning to assess twenty patients (thirteen men and seven women) before and after treatment with paroxetine. The pattern of the scan, they contended, could be used to predict who might benefit from the drug and who would not.[129]

In 2000, a pair of researchers in London, England, tried to distinguish anatomically between two positive emotions – romantic love and friendship – by asking for volunteers, both male and female, who were 'truly, deeply and madly in love' with their partners (of either the same or different sex). The degree to which they were in love was confirmed by a scale established in 1986.[130] The seventeen volunteers selected (eleven women and six men) were shown pictures (which they had supplied) of their lovers and of four friends with whom they were not in love. Their responses were documented by skin galvanic responses and by MRI. The researchers established anatomic sites for romantic love and likened it to euphoric states.[131]

This research is still in its infancy. So few chemicals in the brain are understood. Serotonin and dopamine were the big ones when I went to medical school; to my surprise, they are still important and their actions continue to generate questions. One researcher, who had reviewed the literature on PET scanning and OCD, asked if the areas of increased neurochemical activity necessarily represented the *cause* of the disease. Could they not, in fact, be a *side effect* of, or even a *compensation* for, decreased activity somewhere else? If so, 'treatment' to eliminate those activities might actually be detrimental.[132] And who can confirm that the concentration of a drug in a part of the brain means that it is being 'used' rather than simply residing there? But as we saw in chapter 1, drug companies sponsor research, and the pressure to direct studies into the most obvious channels are great.

Now to bring this rambling example back to love. Is love really localized in the same parts of the brain as OCD? Alas, Henry Dinsdale can no longer find the article he had been reading back in May 1999, and neither can I, although we have identified several possibilities.[133] By that summer, the media began noticing the work of Donatella Marazziti, who chairs the psychiatry group in Pisa, Italy, and of psychologist Cindy Hazan of Cornell University. Marazziti related romantic love to OCD, and Hazan found that normally it lasted only eighteen to thirty months.[134] They both hypothesized ecological arguments about perpetuation of the species to explain their findings. A similar report in March 2002 quoted anthropologist Helen Fisher, who described neuroanatomical experiments being conducted by unnamed researchers at Albert Einstein College of Medicine.[135] She too observed that romantic love endures only a number of months, the time needed to conceive, give birth to, and nurse a child.

But, as Dr Dinsdale said, it should scarcely surprise us if the chemistry of love were to resemble that of OCD. Like obsession, lovesickness was formulated many times in the past as a form of melancholy, a 'monomania,' a delusion over a single object. As one definition would have it, love is an irrational exaggeration, an overvaluing of the marginal differences that exist between one human being and another – a transient delusional state.[136] Psychiatrists have long noticed love's similarity to obsession, which they define as an overwhelming preoccupation with a thing or a behaviour. Why not an overwhelming preoccupation with a person? If love has so many behavioural and emotional features in common with obsession, will it not also share neuroanatomical and neurochemical properties as well?

Now, suppose that love does resemble OCD on scanning of the brain. True, that alone doth not a disease make – no more than discovery of a gene coding for eye colour makes blue eyes a disease. But suppose love, or some *kind* of love is *already* deemed bad, or socially unacceptable, or pathological – like that of women with *DSM* erotomania, or that of the 'impaired therapists' with 'malignant eroticized countertransference.' How long would it be before drug companies conducted trials of medications to solve the problem, using drugs like fluvoxamine and clomipramine that are now employed for OCD? How do we know that these trials are not taking place right now? When would this hypothetical new remedy turn into an off-the-shelf pill for other more ubiquitous love problems that threaten quality and length of life – problems, such as assuaging the pain of being jilted, eliminating the stubborn stain of unrequited love, or dealing with a headstrong daughter who has fallen for a fat biker with back hair, multiple piercings, chains, and a tattoo?

This fascinating new area of research brings the ancient malady to the cutting edge of scientific preoccupation. But it happens only because we are already agreed that, sometimes, love is something bad and, hopefully, discontinuous – a problem needing to be fixed.

Addiction and Psychology: Example 5

If ever we find that new cure for love, my last example would represent a host of prospective consumers: co-dependent women. They are found in the literature on the psychology of addiction. Following the medicalization of the alcoholic from worthless deviant to innocent patient,[137] research turned to the plight of their partners, mostly women, who tolerate and care for them, despite being ignored, if not abused. Like battered wives, they make observers wonder why they do not simply give up on the creep and leave.

To explain this perplexing situation, the idea was born that the addict's partner must derive personal benefit from the relationship. Somehow, she must need her addicted and/or physically or emotionally abusive husband to fill obscure but yawning gaps in her life. The relationship becomes a kind of *folie à deux*: the addict persists in using, the partner consoles herself in the role of his supporter. The concept was embraced by many women because it offered several advantages. For a change, it focused attention on someone who was too easily and too often overlooked. It relieved feelings of weakness and duplicity. The seemingly self-destructive behaviour became an excessive, almost noble, 'need to nurture,' the natural product of a warped upbringing. Above all, it absolved guilt: neither her behaviour (nor his, for that matter) were her fault. These benefits provided a market.

The history of this disease has just begun to be written, partly because it is new and controversial; as one writer put it, 'its robustness is open to challenge.'[138] Co-dependency as a concept originated in the late 1970s, in the twelve-step programs of Alcoholics Anonymous devoted to the so-called 'alcoholic family.' In the mid-1980s, it was boosted by soothing popular literature for 'misunderstood' and 'mistreated' women who simply (and euphemistically) 'love too much.'[139] Later it was embraced by some doctors, who gave it diagnostic criteria and placed it in the *DSM* as a type of dependent personality disorder.[140] It has been a Medical Subject Heading on Medline since 1992.

Attractive accounts of co-dependency emphasize the illness:

'symptoms' of strong nurturing and coping skills in people who otherwise lack self-confidence.[141] Less attractive accounts focus on the co-dependant's manipulative narcissism and self-destructive weakness.[142] Scales have been made to measure co-dependency, and studies estimate as many as forty million co-dependent people in the United States.[143] Because co-dependency pathologizes traditionally feminine characteristics, it may be mirrored by folk diseases in other cultures.[144]

Much of the debate over co-dependency takes place in the nursing literature by a delicious extrapolation of fuzzy logic. Nurses nurture. If co-dependency means an increased urge to nurture, then maybe all nurturers – or the really good ones – are co-dependants. Sides are chosen by those who are willing, if not relieved, to discover that they are sick[145] and by those who wish to distance themselves as far as possible from that notion.[146]

But what is a co-dependent, if not a lover – so loyal in her love that she abides an abuser who would repel anyone else? She stands by her man. She keeps her vows to the letter – for richer or poorer, in sickness and health, for better or worse (especially worse) – until her death, a death frequently hastened by the poverty, sickness, and very danger of her love. Co-dependency is yet another name for lovesickness.

Conclusion: On the Badness of Love

In this chapter, I have shown that

- love was considered a disease for centuries;
- lovesickness originated in society, not medicine, and was first described by artists, then much later by doctors;
- once medicalized, science was invoked to explain and treat love;
- in every era, lovesickness respected vogue in philosophy and science;

- lovesickness seemed to wane after 1900;
- cultural doubt remains about the goodness of love; and
- sometimes, love is still a disease.

The question is, why is love still a disease? Remember that disease formulations in the West conform to the medical model and the organismic theory. They insist that the disease resides in an individual and that it is bad or undesirable. These assumptions go with the organismic theory. The story of lovesickness demonstrates the power of sociocultural preconvictions in deciding when something is bad enough to be a sickness. It also shows the power of the philosophical method of disease construction itself: in each time and place, the problem was made to fit the pattern of what every well-dressed disease must wear, both scientifically and philosophically.[147]

With lovesickness, we betray our utter slavery to the organismic idea that disease must affect an individual. Take for example, the medicalization of co-dependency or that of the battered wife. Were we able to contemplate sickness in populations, we might pathologize the collective, social ills that create and tolerate substance abuse, domestic violence, and sports thugs.[148] The pretty young women in plate 2.6 came out in support of the famous hockey hero who was charged with assault against another player; will any of them end up with a diagnosis of co-dependent personality?[149] And yet, why should women who support their partners be considered sick when it is our society that glorifies violence, that revels in hockey fights, that sees 'head-bashing' in sport as 'normal' if not entertaining, that displays thousands of television murders each year, and that teaches little boys to be manly by finding solutions with their fists? The literature on these problems can be found in sociology not medicine.[150] Could a nonorganismic or population theory be a more appropriate way to medicalize the problem of the unfortunate woman *and* her addicted partner? If so, our whole society

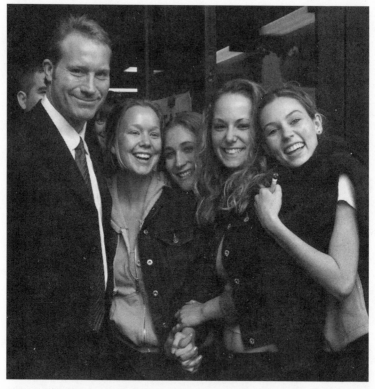

Plate 2.6 Marty McSorley with young admirers ('Slash, head bash normal ...,' *Globe and Mail*, 29 September 2000, A14).

would be seen as sick for tolerating and sometimes celebrating male violence and for creating conditions that lead to addiction. Without contemplating the role of society, how can medicine find ways to prevent co-dependency? Does it not make more sense to try to prevent abuse rather than to cure love?

As for 'bad,' what prompts our society and so many others in the past to accept the pathologization of something so beautiful and exhilarating as that unique, pleasurable bond with another human being? Why are we threatened by lovers?

It is not sex. Perhaps for a while, the physical side of love added to the mistrust, especially in the Reformation and maybe again in the nineteenth century with its determined focus on organs. But that was not the case for most of time, and it is certainly not the case now. Sex is flaunted and cherished; if sex is 'broken,' doctors and drug companies are summoned to fix it.

I think love is threatening because it promises loss of control. In putting someone else ahead of herself, a lover embraces risks – in the mild sense, of being laughed at, rejected, or losing face. In a stronger sense, she risks loss of her personal freedom with the headlong impulse to commit forever and ever. In the extreme sense, she risks her existence. These dangerous 'choices' could be detrimental to individual autonomy, health, and life.[151] The affront does not stop there: it extends to the rest of society. In finding a unique, private happiness, alone and apart, successful lovers place their union above everyone and everything. The rest of society comforts itself with controls both secular and religious: customs, regulations, and licences for engagement, marriage, and divorce; laws to specify who may and may not apply.[152] Even as I write in the wake of the Ontario court decision that followed these lectures, some sectors of society fret over allowing marriage between lovers of the same sex. Much like Ludwik Fleck's observation about illness and tainted blood, this mistrust of love is a primordial doubt that pervades our culture. The Greeks knew it, and they told us: Eros was born of Chaos, and his arrows could carry us back whence he came.

Love is a siren that lures and tempts us at every turn, and all indicators suggest that love can still be a disease.

3

Livers: The Rise of Hepatitis C

Mr R. lay rigidly on the examining table staring up at the ceiling and rehearsing his complaints in an aggravated monotone. The seventy-six-year-old was grief stricken over the sudden death of his married daughter just six months earlier. Children are not supposed to disappear before their parents. He was back for a check-up of his polycythemia rubra vera (PRV), a slowly malignant condition of bone marrow, characterized by production of too many red blood cells. We still get to use the ancient method of bleeding to treat people with PRV. After two decades, however, Mr R's disease was in the burnout stage, and he no longer needed treatment. To be frank, blood was the least of his problems. Mr R was a walking medical miracle. His first heart attack had been back in 1966 when he was only forty-three years old. At age sixty-three, he had survived coronary bypass surgery, which had cured his angina and the heart attacks, but he now had a huge aortic aneurysm. Although a surgeon was willing to repair it, the anesthetists advised against an operation because of his cardiac history. The state of his lower legs and feet indicated that his smaller blood vessels were in rough shape too; nothing surgical could be done for them. It might help if he quit smoking, but given his age and his psychological misery, that seemed unlikely. Mr R's liver function was completely normal, but he had learned that his blood was positive for hepatitis C. The source was presumed to be the transfusions he'd received during his heart surgery thirteen years ago.

'It's ridiculous,' he muttered. '$10,000! It's nothing for an entire life.'

'What?' I asked unplugging my stethoscope from my ears and my attention from his repaired heart.

'Nothing!' he said. 'Typical of those government bug-
gers to think they can buy us off with a cash handout like
that. My whole life is destroyed. Ten thousand is nothing.
It's an insult.'

Foolishly, I tried to remonstrate.

'But Mr R! Your liver is fine, and it stands a good
chance of staying fine for a long time! You've got a lot of
other problems and you might not even be here now if
you hadn't had that operation on your heart.'

He would not be dissuaded: he had hepatitis C, and it
would kill him. His only symptom from this new diagnosis was anger.

The liver is a majestic organ – stolidly culinary, anatomically
obscure, and magically indispensable (plate 3.1). We know it has
something to do with digestion, drinking, and blood. In Quebec, 'le foie' substitutes for the gallbladder; in France, 'une crise
de foie' is a metaphor for general disarray. The history of liver
disease could follow many avenues; in this chapter, we will
focus on just one: hepatitis. Following the report of audience
participation, we will quickly review the long trajectory of hepatitis from the elegant descriptions of the ancients to the recognition and rise of hepatitis C in our own time. Once again, the
concepts described in the first chapter will assist in the analysis.
In conclusion, I will unite my observations about livers with
those I made in the two previous chapters about disease concepts in general and about lovers in particular.

Hepatitis poses no exception to the general theme that we
have been exploring: disease constructs emerge from social as
well as biological conventions, and they are constantly revised
to fit moral and intellectual premises. A single disease type for
many centuries, the hepatitides (now plural) multiplied out of
an explanatory problem generated by clinical observations,
advances in science, and political events. Hepatitis C is a dis-

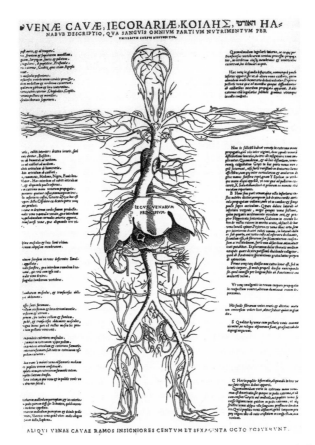

Plate 3.1 The liver and veins, detail from Andreas Vesalius, *Tabulae anatomicae sex*, 1538.

tinct new disease. Suspected long before the 'discovery' of its virus was announced in 1989, it is still under construction. In a sense, hepatitis C represents one of several conceptual splittings, a hiving off from a traditional monolith of liver ailments. Many of its causes and some – though far from all – of its symptoms, like those of Mr R, emerge from social perceptions. They will defy scientific reduction for years to come.

Audience Participation: Whither Jaundice?

On the evening of the last lecture, I asked members of the audience if they could remember a disease called 'the jaundice,' sometimes expressed in the charmingly redundant form, 'yellow jaundice.' I was not looking for comprehension of the words, but for recollection of a time when people used to catch jaundice. I suspected that memory of this ailment would be confined to people who were born before 1955. To test that theory I asked members of the audience for anonymous written responses – 'yes' (I remember) or 'no' (I do not) – together with their year of birth. I also asked for information about personal experiences with hepatitis or jaundice in themselves or others. The responses seemed to confirm my theory (see table 3.1).

Table 3.1 Familiarity with '[yellow] jaundice' and hepatitis, by age, London Ontario, October 2002

Birth	Recollection of jaundice (%)	Personal experience of jaundice or hepatitis (%)
Before 1940	100	20
1940–9	62.5	25
1950–9	66	33
1960–9	33	0
1970–9	0	42.8
After 1980	0	0

The results confirm that familiarity with the diagnosis of 'yellow jaundice' declined and vanished after the 1960s. Nevertheless, personal familiarity with hepatitis continues at a steadily variable rate; it is intriguing that the greatest personal contact with 'hepatitis' is in a group of people now in their late twenties and early thirties, none of whom recall 'jaundice' as a diagnosis. This exercise provides another demonstration of the continuity of illness in the face of changing disease names or diagnoses.

Early Descriptions of Hepatitis, or When Did the Liver Inflame?

The jaundice of the 1940s and 1950s went something like this: a disease, situated in the liver, characterized by general malaise, loss of appetite, chills, fever, pain in the right upper abdomen and sometimes in the right shoulder. Increasing yellowness of the skin and, especially, the eyes, dark urine, pale stools, and intense itching proportional to the degree of yellowness, and aversion to smoking (if the patient was a smoker). The liver and the spleen could be enlarged, and the white blood cell count elevated. Extreme cases featured drowsiness, hiccups, swelling of the abdomen with ascites fluid, vomiting of blood, and other bleeding; an abscess could form in the liver, and the kidneys might fail. Jaundice might occur in isolation, or following injuries and acute diseases of other organs, such as pneumonia, malaria, and bowel disease. In newborns, jaundice could cause kernicterus, or permanent brain damage. When occurring in clusters, jaundice appeared to be contagious; often, it was fatal. Then as now, cures were unknown, but helpful measures included rest, fluids, surgical drainage of abscesses, and quarantine.

This entire description – minus only the references to smoking, mental retardation, and quarantine – is nearly identical to that of Hippocrates 2500 years ago. Granted the words 'white blood cell count' were not used by the ancients, but the Hippocratic author noticed the same phenomenon in a thick 'buffy' layer that developed over the surface of the patient's blood after it had been let; he called it 'leucophlegmasia,' which means an increase in the white part of the blood.[1]

'Hepatitis' is described in at least seven different treatises of the Hippocratic Corpus, one of the fullest descriptions being in *Internal Affections*, translated by Paul Potter of the University of Western Ontario.[2] Yellowness tending to green, or jaundice –

'jaunesse' in French – was the cardinal symptom. The Hippocratic writers related the outcome to the intensity or shade of the
colour; without exception, they situated jaundice in the liver.
The physiological theory of the ancients was that black bile had
accumulated in the liver, blocking the yellow bile normally produced there, and causing it to spill over into the rest of the body.

The rich clinical observations of the Hippocratics were amplified in the second century AD by Aretaeus of Cappadocia, who
wrote about hepatitis in all four of his extant treatises and
explained the symptoms with anatomy and physiology. Loss of
appetite occurred, he wrote, because food tasted bitter 'for the
bile is the screen of fallacious tastes.'[3] The patient had a tendency to bleed: first, because varices (dilated veins) grew
around the portal vein,[4] and second, because the liver's 'power
of nutrition'[5] was weakened, meaning it could not form blood
and bile as usual.[6]

Aretaeus recognized several different types of hepatitis. Like
Hippocrates, he distinguished them by variations in colour
and also by organic origin and clinical patterns. The disease
stemmed from 'intemperance,'[7] he said, and from afflictions of
other organs.[8] As for prognosis, jaundice caused by obstructed
bile ducts without inflammation was not dangerous 'for the
liver is not disordered';[9] however, 'with inflammation [of the
liver],' jaundice proves fatal and 'terminates most commonly in
dropsy [or swelling] and cachexia [or wasting]. And many have
died emaciated, without dropsy.'[10]

Twenty to twenty-five centuries later, these descriptions are
astonishingly precise. Jaundice must have been common for the
ancients to have gathered such a wealth of clinical experience.
They were more optimistic about treatment than we are now,
advocating frankincense, aloes, and bleeding to evacuate the
noxious black bile.

Aretaeus's comments about danger of inflammation are especially interesting. The Greek word used in these descriptions

was always 'hepatitis.' In the nineteenth century, Emile Littré, the French scholar whose ten-volume Hippocrates remains a standard reference work, translated occurrences of the Greek word 'hepatitis' as 'hépatite.'[11] In today's medical terminology, any word with the suffix '-itis' represents 'inflammation.' The classic description of inflammation is generally ascribed to the first-century Roman physician Celsus, whose words are oft-cited in Latin by modern pathologists and clinicians wishing to flash their erudition: 'rubor, dolor, calor, tumor, et laesio functione' (redness, pain, heat, swelling, and loss of function). Nowadays, inflammation is suspected in the clinical setting and confirmed in the laboratory under the microscope. But there were no microscopes in antiquity. Did 'hepatitis' mean the same thing then as it does now? Littré's successor (and our colleague), Paul Potter, translated 'hepatitis' more cautiously as 'a disease of the liver.'[12]

It was not until the eighteenth century, with the work of François Boissier de Sauvages, that the meaning of words ending in '-itis' was restricted to inflammation.[13] We met Sauvages in the last chapter as the eighteen-year-old author of a Montpellier thesis on lovesickness. The Greek word 'hepatitis' is a 'fausse ami,' which will lead us astray if we think it meant the same thing in the past as it does now. To translate it into English as 'hepatitis' would bestow on it a pathophysiologic meaning that it did not possess in antiquity. 'Hepatitis' for Hippocrates and Aretaeus meant *any* disease of the liver, usually associated with jaundice. Professor Potter's translation comes at the expense of having to alter a word that ostensibly needed no change, but it avoids anachronistic imputing of modern concepts to ancient words.

Indeed, the broader interpretation makes good sense even to a nonphilologist like me. If we go back to the ancient writings, applying the scorned but seductively attractive lens of the 'retrospectoscope,' we observe that these descriptions apply equally well to conditions *other* than present-day hepatitis: including noninflammatory problems of the liver, such as cirrhosis and metastatic cancer, and problems external to the liver, such as hemolytic anemia, gallbladder stones, or pancreatic tumour. The nuances embedded in these interpretations can only deepen our respect for the ancients who so closely observed the sufferings of their patients, considered them carefully, set them into a framework consistent with their scientific knowledge, and wrote it all down.

To make a quick end of this overview of the long history of hepatitis: no one improved these ancient descriptions for two thousand years.

Liver under the Microscope: Hepatitis Stands Alone

Hepatitis was teased out of a tangled morass of liver ailments, first linguistically with the precisions attached to the suffix '-itis' (restricting it to inflammation), and then, pathologically with the advent of autopsy, microscopy, cell theory, and biochemistry. In some ways, hepatitis was always 'left over,' as other types of liver disease left the morass to become their own distinct entities. The nineteenth and early twentieth centuries saw the elaboration of hepatic cancer,[14] cirrhosis,[15] leukemia,[16] Budd Chiari syndrome,[17] lipid storage diseases,[18] parasitic infections,[19] the myeloproliferative diseases,[20] porphyria,[21] thalassemia,[22] favism,[23] hemolytic anemias, and various liver toxicities. 'Hepatitis' was what remained with its mysterious array of apparent causes, its variable course, and its stubborn refusal to be cured by art.

Within the category of hepatitis, clinical distinctions emerged. Some hepatitis was considered infectious, especially when it occurred in epidemic clusters.[24] Patterns of symptoms and recovery could vary. A few cases were 'fulminant' or rapidly fatal. In particular, yellow fever was recognized as a distinct and severe form of epidemic hepatitis. It ravaged pre-Columbian

Central America; however, with a few suggestive exceptions, it seems not to have existed in Europe until it was introduced in modern times. The distinctive clinical manifestations of yellow fever were described following several devastating outbreaks that killed more than 100,000 Americans from the seventeenth to the twentieth centuries.[25] Soon after the advent of germ theory, a search for bacterial causes of liver ailments failed. In 1900, however, great excitement greeted Walter Reed's announcement that yellow fever was caused by a virus and transmitted by a mosquito vector. In the developed world, control of this dreaded form of hepatitis followed quickly, first by mechanical prevention and later by vaccine.[26] Yellow fever is still endemic in sub-Saharan Africa and parts of South America, where case fatality is as high as 65 per cent.

Yet more hepatitis remained. Most cases healed spontaneously, but death could occur. What determined the fluctuations in virulence and severity was not clear. By the mid-twentieth century, when a certain comfort level had developed with the technique of liver biopsy – either through a needle or an open incision[27] – physicians realized that the after-effects of even a mild attack of hepatitis could endure for years as continuous low-grade inflammation. Scar tissue, cirrhosis, and tumours could be the late result. The terms 'chronic active hepatitis' and 'cryptogenic cirrhosis' were developed to express (if not explain) the mystery of persistent inflammation in the liver and/or the advent of cirrhosis following a bout of 'subclinical' hepatitis that had passed unnoticed – even by the patient.

Doctors were stumped. Nothing would allow for a meaningful separation of the myriad clinical manifestations of this disease.

Hepatitis and Blood

In 1943, Paul Beeson noticed that hepatitis sometimes occurred one to four months after blood transfusion.[28] Four decades had elapsed since Karl Landsteiner made his important observations about blood groups that were to form the basis of transfusion medicine. Why did it take so long for someone to link blood transfusions with liver disease? First, transfusion had been used only sparingly and in dire situations; Landsteiner did not receive his Nobel prize until 1930, when transfusion was becoming a frequent peacetime practice. Beeson's research came a mere decade later. Second, it took a long time to make the connection because it could take up to four months for the symptoms of post-transfusion hepatitis to develop, plenty of time for the transfusion event to have been forgotten or discounted.

After 1943, hepatitis was sorted clinically – that is by its mode of transmission – into two disease types: 'infectious' hepatitis and 'serum' hepatitis. 'Infectious' hepatitis was spread easily by fecal-oral contamination; 'serum' hepatitis could be transmitted only by mixing of body fluids. Both could be fatal, but serum hepatitis seemed to be more dangerous. These two distinctions within a single disease entity implied that two different viruses could cause it; however, those 'causes' were merely presumed to be different. It was not the cause but the *route* of infection that provided the basis for the diagnostic distinction.

These new scientific terms, 'serum' and 'infectious' hepatitis, were added to the lay expression (yellow) 'jaundice,' recalled by older members of the Goodman audience. Instead of describing symptoms or tissue pathology, these new names hinted at a cause, or at least at the route of infection. They would stand for the next twenty years during a fascinating period of medical investigation that inevitably shaped their demise. Their adoption conveyed several implications, three of which are described below.

First, the clinical picture was refined. Incubation periods could now be measured and compared. Serum hepatitis seemed to have a longer incubation period, suggesting that the causative agents had to be at least two different viruses. Subclinical infections were captured and monitored for prevalence and subtle manifestations. The infamous Willowbrook study, often portrayed as one of the most unethical experiments of modern times, addressed these preoccupations. In that trial, published in 1967 by Saul Krugman of New York, mentally retarded children, newly admitted to the overcrowded Willowbrook state institution on Staten Island, were deliberately fed or injected with infected fluids. They were isolated from the other residents while waiting for symptoms or signs to appear, be measured, and monitored. Krugman's team had obtained parental permission, but some argue that consent had been coerced with the promise of admitting the child to the institution in exchange for participation in the study. The researchers justified their approach with the observation that hygiene was impossible to maintain and all the children would eventually be exposed to hepatitis anyway, possibly dying from it.[29] Their work took place in the aftermath of a devastating measles epidemic that had claimed the lives of sixty children in the same institution, and a high priority was placed on avoiding another deadly outbreak. This justification was considered adequate by the scientific establishment and by Krugman himself, but it was questioned in the leading journals. It still carries no weight with some bioethicists, lawyers, and suspicious patient-support groups that now liken Krugman's research to that of Nazi doctors.[30] Nevertheless, Krugman has received many prestigious awards, and his name adorns a festschrift, a lectureship, and an infectious disease unit.

Second – and recalling our disease 'triangle' from the first chapter – anticipated sufferers took on special identities or 'types' that became part of the disease concept. Infectious hepatitis affected the poverty stricken, the lax, the institutionalized, and the unclean; it was a disease of beatniks, 'street people,' and 'hippies.'[31] Those likely to develop serum hepatitis were a mélange of the 'guilty' – self mutilators and needle-sharing drug users – and of the 'innocent' – recipients of blood or the heroic nurses and surgeons who had cared for them.

Third, the knowledge that blood transfusion could cause hepatitis (in addition to syphilis, malaria, and other infections) was disturbing. The more exposure to blood, the greater the chances of infection. Hepatitis must join the long and growing list of iatrogenic diseases, which are the health problems caused by doctors. One 1959 study showed that hepatitis followed 17 to 100 per cent of transfusions.[32] Finding a way to test donor blood for hepatitis was imperative. People who had ever suffered from jaundice were asked not to donate. The limitations of this control measure were obvious from the outset; physicians already understood that some well-intentioned donors carried hepatitis without knowing it. What else was to be done? Doctors were urged to use blood sparingly.

But the pressure to transfuse was great. The 1960s and early 1970s saw exciting new developments in cardiovascular surgery, plastic surgery, renal dialysis, transplantation, and hematology, all of which relied on an ample blood supply. The heart-lung bypass consumed several donor units simply to prime the machine. For the anesthetist who monitored a falling blood pressure at the end of a lengthy operation, or for the nephrologist whose tired dialysis patient had a hemoglobin less than a third of her own, nothing seemed easier, safer, or more reasonable than hanging another bag of packed cells. The benefits were instantaneous; the harm, invisible.

Alphabetical Hepatitis: A, B, C, D, E ... or Not

In that fruitful period of scientific endeavour while elective surgeries increased, the need to protect the blood supply loomed larger, and hepatitis moved into the realm of immunology and virology. Research began to focus on how to identify those who could spread the disease but had never felt sick.

All were agreed that a virus, possibly more than one, had to be involved. Viruses were difficult to see; only with electron microscopy, invented in 1931, had they actually become visible. Nevertheless, viruses did not have to be seen to be detected and controlled. Scientists had hypothesized their existence long before they could see them. Viruses represented infective matter that could pass through a filter which would normally block larger bacteria. They could also be detected by the immune responses that they provoked in living creatures – chemical reactions between antigens (from viruses) and antibodies (immune reactors from infected animals). A vaccine causes an animal to make lots of antibodies (hopefully) without making it sick. Several successful vaccines had already been produced against what are now known to be viral illnesses. For example, in the late eighteenth century, Edward Jenner had used vaccinia virus (cowpox) to prevent infection with variola virus (small-pox). In similar ways, rabies, yellow fever, and polio had already been tamed by the mid-twentieth century.

Virology was cutting-edge science. In 1951 the Nobel prize went to Max Theiler for his work on yellow fever virus and vaccine. Three years later, it went to the team of John F. Enders, Frederick Chapman Robbins, and Thomas Huckle Weller, who had cultured polio virus (rather than to either Jonas Salk or Albert Bruce Sabin, who developed vaccines). If the cause of hepatitis was indeed a virus, researchers had several distinguished models to use as guides.

The first virological successes in hepatitis research came with Baruch Blumberg's 1965 discovery of the Australian antigen. It was a protein in the blood of a hemophiliac whose blood reacted with that of an Australian aborigine whom he had never met. The hypothesis was that because of his multiple transfusions, the hemophiliac had made an antibody to something that was carried in the blood of at least one of his donors and in the blood of the aborigine. A similar protein was found in the blood of leukemics who had also been multiply transfused. By 1968, Blumberg had linked the Australian antigen to serum hepatitis using studies on asymptomatic children with trisomy-21 (Down syndrome).[33]

Australian antigen was big news. It was thought to be a piece of the virus that caused serum hepatitis, but exactly which part would not be clear for a long time. Several other pieces were soon found. An antibody to Australian antigen was produced and a test was developed to identify carriers of the antigen in order to protect the blood supply from hepatitis.[34] This test was applied to all blood products in Canada by 1972. Transfusion experts, hepatologists, and surgeons were ecstatic. Blumberg shared the Nobel prize in 1976. Work on a vaccine was soon underway, and trials began in 1979.[35] Still characterized by yellowness in its most severe forms, hepatitis again went through a name change. The kind of hepatitis that had previously been called 'infectious' or 'hippie' was now called 'hepatitis A,' while the term 'serum hepatitis' faded in 1981 to be replaced by 'hepatitis B.'

The Australian antigen test for hepatitis B also confirmed what transfusion agencies had suspected since at least 1959: paid donors were much more likely to carry hepatitis B than volunteers.[36] People who needed to sell their blood were more often those whose poverty was associated with risky practices such as prostitution or illegal intravenous drug use. Canada did not use paid donors and its incidence of infection was thought to be lower, but no studies were done. The United States did use bought blood, allowing it to be distributed together with donations from volunteers.[37] Post-transfusion hepatitis was thought to occur in as many as 33 per cent of heart surgery patients who would have received many units of blood.[38] Without the paid donors, providers argued, demand for blood would exceed supply. In the absence of reliable screening tests, the epidemiological implications could be easily downplayed.

After hepatitis B screening became available, the long-held suspicions were confirmed when the group of paid donors was shown to be highly infective for that one disease.[39] Concerns were then raised about all the other undetectable infections that might still be lurking in bought blood. Repeated calls for the elimination of payment met with resistance. A small but significant victory was won in 1976 when the American Food and Drug Administration required blood banks to label products from paid donors. The market quickly decided the future: clinicians avoided bought blood, and the system shifted to volunteers.[40] Paid donors with special blood types are still used for cytapheresis products in the United States and Canada for the collection of specific components – not without controversy.[41]

The excitement over hepatitis B testing quickly turned to disappointment. Post-transfusion hepatitis soon revealed itself to be much more complicated than the A and B classification had implied. The picture was further clouded by the nearly simultaneous banishing of paid donors. All donor blood was now tested for the Australian antigen, but less than half – perhaps only 25 per cent – of post-transfusion hepatitis was eliminated by this screening for hepatitis B (figure 3.1).[42] Perhaps hepatitis A would account for the remainder, although its virus had yet to be identified.

In the scramble to find the culprit responsible for remaining transfusion-related hepatitis, Stephen Feinstone and his team at the National Institutes of Health (NIH) examined hundreds of infected stool samples with electron microscopy. Once they had found a likely virus for hepatitis A, they experimented on themselves to prove that it was the right bug. They announced success in 1973.[43] Soon, however, more disappointment ensued: hepatitis A virus caused none of the unexplained cases of post-transfusion hepatitis; it was a separate disease, clinically and virologically.[44] The clinical distinctions of Saul Krugman were vindicated.

Figure 3.1 Incidence of post-transfusion hepatitis in the United States

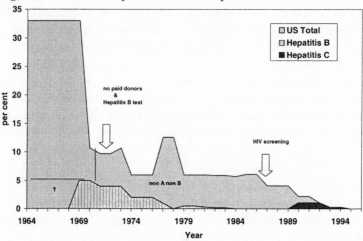

Source: Based on Alter, 2000

Nevertheless, those persistent clinical distinctions posed a problem: they were based on presumed differences in the *routes* of infection, but both diseases had always been 'infectious,' and now even the *routes* of infection as well as the cause had begun to blur. In 1975–6, ending several years of speculation, German, British, and American scientists demonstrated that serum hepatitis could be spread sexually.[45] Working out the venereal epidemiology of hepatitis B and conducting trials with its vaccine relied on the generous cooperation of gay organizations in New York, Seattle, San Francisco, and other major cities.[46] These loose networks readily revived when they were called upon to study AIDS just a few years later. The bewildering array of vehicles that can convey hepatitis B infection continues to diversify and now ranges from thorn bushes to suicide bombers.[47]

By late 1975, scientists had to admit at least one of two discouraging things: either their tests were too feeble to detect all hepatitis B infections, or at least one other unknown virus was involved in most post-transfusion hepatitis.[48] This new but once again 'leftover' hepatitis was referred to, somewhat clumsily, as 'hepatitis non-A non-B.'[49] The disease was of unknown cause – just as all hepatitis had been for the preceding two millennia. It affected, but was not confined to, people who had been transfused. It was carried by thousands of apparently healthy donors. Hepatitis C would emerge from hepatitis non-A non-B, but not until fifteen more years had passed, much longer than anyone expected.

Most histories of hepatitis C choose to begin at this moment.[50] While hepatitis non-A non-B was being defined, at least four other hepatitis viruses were identified, one of which has been cloned – hepatitis D, E (cloned in 1990), F, and G – each creating a separate disease, with its own clinical pattern.[51] The diagnosis had little to do with yellowness (jaundice), although the symptom remained as a possibility. The diagnosis now depended on demonstrating the presence of liver dysfunction or a specific virus, whether or not the patient had any symptoms at all. With reference to the Hippocratic triangle of chapter 1, the importance of the illness in the concept of hepatitis waned, while that of the observer grew.

During this period, restrictions on the use of blood were urged by hospitals, hematologists, gastroenterologists, and surgeons. As a medical student in the early 1970s, I was taught that a blood transfusion is 'a potentially life-threatening intervention,' resorted to only when the risks of not using it were obvious and great.[52] I graduated in 1974, the year that hepatitis non-A non-B was first postulated. In hematology, we were vigilant never to transfuse lightly. But blood was useful and it was seductive.

The Failure of Prevention through Control: Two Memories

I have two vivid memories of the built-in conflicts surrounding blood use from my days as a resident in Toronto.

Memory One

In 1965, a method was found to concentrate the clotting factors of blood that were needed by hemophiliacs.[53] Called cryoprecipitate, the product revolutionized the quality and length of life for many bleeders. 'Cryo' was kept frozen in tiny bags, each representing the quantity of factor VIII obtained from a single donation. If a hemophiliac had a bleed, or was going to have an operation, six to twelve of the little bags were floated in warm water to thaw; their contents were then drawn into a syringe and injected into the patient. Some centres allowed hemophiliacs to keep cryoprecipitate at home for administration by themselves or family members; the Toronto hospital where I worked did not. The patient with a bleed had to rush to the hospital and wait for the resident to show up. If the young man was over the age of ten, he was only too familiar with the routine and had formed strong views about what was wrong with the health care system and which residents were dolts, and he had no hesitation about airing them. From multiple transfusions in his past, he also had scarred veins, making the injection painful for him and for his attendants. Hemophiliacs were notoriously more adept at puncturing their own elusive vessels with a needle than any callow member of the house staff.

One evening in 1979, I was summoned to administer cryoprecipitate to 'John,' a young student in his first year of university. Slight, with long hair, he exuded the funky appeal of a budding artist. He was nice enough to me as I fumbled with the water, bags, tubing, and gigantic syringe, but he fumed about having to be there at all and kept up a *basso continuo* of grievances. Instead of 'cryo,' he wanted to use lyophilized factor VIII concentrate. It was a powder that did not need to be refrigerated; it could be reconstituted simply by adding sterile fluid to a small bottle. Above all, from his perspective, it could be taken camping. He slipped into a polemic that had clearly been rehearsed.

Never had he been allowed to take a holiday more than an hour or two from the hospital freezer. Did I have any idea what it meant not to be able to go on a canoe trip? Or how stigmatizing that deprivation must be for a Canadian male? What right did we have to keep John from being normal, when science had already made it possible for him to do everything his friends could do?

Foolishly, I tried to remonstrate. I had read of those new products too, and as a well-indoctrinated resident, I had absorbed the reasons why we were not using them. It was a problem of method. To freeze-dry the precious factors, thousands of units of blood had to be pooled. If just one of those units had hepatitis, then all doses in all the bottles made from that pool would have hepatitis. Even with hepatitis B screening, lots of other non-A non-B hepatitis was getting through. We already had a similar situation for patients with factor IX deficiency, or Christmas disease. Their replacement factor could be obtained *only* in pooled product. A large percentage of those young men developed hepatitis before they turned twenty. John's dose of 'cryo' represented the blood of only a few people; lyophilized factor represented blood from thousands. Was it a good idea to let him run an even greater risk of hepatitis simply to go on a canoe trip?

I could tell that my argument was unconvincing. He wasn't having any of it and retorted, quick as lightning, that the entire medical profession was paternalistic, interested only in control. I was turning out to be a good doctor, he said, because I was just as bad as all the others. I gave him the 'cryo.' Drawing himself up with great dignity as he drew his sleeve down, he asked, 'Why can't you let me decide about my own risks?' Irrefutable logic expressed by the confident immortality of youth.

The fretting medics lost this battle for control soon after. Lyophilized factor concentrates became widely used, and the tragic results are well known. Less than four years later, in January

1983, an editorial in the *New England Journal* urged that hemophiliacs be treated with cryoprecipitate instead of lyophilized concentrate.[54] I cannot remember the young man's real name, but I have always wondered what happened to him. Given the date of our conversation and the severity of his problem, he had a 70 per cent chance of being infected with HIV within those four years;[55] he had a 50 per cent chance of being dead of AIDS or hepatitis (or both) before he was thirty.[56]

I hope he got to go on a canoe trip.

Memory Two

This memory is also about control of blood products. For some reason, not well understood at the time, lyophilized factor IX had a miraculous effect on cerebral hemorrhages, especially those associated with anticoagulants. But, as I just explained, it carried an extremely high risk of hepatitis because it was made from pooled plasma.[57] We were taught that using factor IX was tantamount to injecting hepatitis. The hematologists at another Toronto hospital put stringent controls on the use of factor IX concentrate: any order sent to the blood bank had to be approved by the resident on call before the product would be released. No one had explained this local peculiarity to me as I joined the hematology team in that hospital. Late one night, in my role as resident on call, I found myself on the telephone with an irate neurosurgeon who was screaming unrepeatable, foul-mouthed invective because he wanted the restricted factor IX for a woman who was lying on the operating table waiting for her intracranial bleeding to be controlled. The gist of his message was that he (godlike neurosurgeon) should not be subjected to the delay and indignity of a frivolous formality to seek approval from me (peon-like, know-nothing resident who couldn't tell a scalpel from a pen). He was calling from the blood bank, where he had gone to demand instant satisfaction. I felt sorry for the technologist, who, I imagined, must be dangling by his necktie from one of the god's rubber-gloved hands while the other grasped the phone.

Foolishly, I tried to remonstrate, if only to explain why such a rule was in place. Big mistake! The response was terrifying. I caved instantly and acquiesced to the surgeon's wish. The next morning I went to the blood bank to see how they were taking it and if anyone needed stitches. 'Oh that's okay,' they said. 'He does that every time he gets a patient with a bleed.' I considered getting a tattoo across my chest saying in large letters 'IF FOUND UNCONSCIOUS, DO NOT TAKE TO HOSPITAL X,' but I worried that the tattoo might give me hepatitis.

These two memories illustrate how difficult it was to prevent transfusion hepatitis back in those days, even when we tried. I left full-time hematology in 1988. If *I* have such memories, think how many more are shared by my clinical colleagues who remained in practice. The deplorable us-versus-them mentality that came later depresses me and distorts history. The worst moment came in the mid-1990s while I was watching a CBC television news report from Parliament Hill in which an angry but seemingly hale protester complained that he had contracted hepatitis from 'a routine blood transfusion.' From our point of view, no blood transfusion was ever 'routine.' Strong pressure to use dangerous products came from the articulate patients themselves and their doctors. But it seems disrespectful to say so, because we are still alive and so many of them are now dead. Yes, it was wrong to let them win. How will we recognize the next time that it will be right to play the part of paternalistic control freaks and withhold a new product against the wishes of patients?

Hepatitis Non-A Non-B and AIDS

What happened next, as everyone knows, was AIDS.[58] It had a profound effect on hepatitis. Coming out of the blue, AIDS seemed much worse than hepatitis – frightening because of its newness, its grotesque effects, its fatal outcome, its transmission through sex and blood, and its seemingly personalized attack on certain social groups. AIDS research displaced hepatitis research. The human immunodeficiency virus (HIV) was found in 1983 – less than three years after the disease first appeared, but at the time, the search seemed to take forever. The democratic and litigious chapters of AIDS history served as a model for hepatitis, and the histories of these two diseases are intertwined. As yet another viral disease spread by transfusion and sex, AIDS infused hepatitis with the same cachet, dragging it into the limelight and the charged rhetoric of guilt and blame.

Blame is a big issue with AIDS. When it first came along patients were blamed. It was seen as a punishment for 'bad behaviours' – homosexuality, drug use, promiscuity. AIDS patients were divided into the innocent and guilty. Those who were infected by transfusions, by their mothers, or by their married partners, were 'innocent victims.' But the implication of this epithet is that all the others were somehow 'guilty' or deserving of their affliction because of who they were or what they did. Yet the suffering was no less. The inequity of these stereotypes was decried in the popular press and the medical literature. Gradually the patient-blaming subsided. Among its many long-term side effects, AIDS taught us to be more tolerant and more vigilant.

But blaming did not go away altogether; rather, it was shifted from the patients to the establishment. Goaded by the litigious models available in the United States, people who had contracted HIV from blood transfusions organized to lobby for more research, to seek out those who were responsible for their infections, and to demand compensation.

Some countries came through quickly with financial help for people infected with AIDS through blood. England was first in March 1988, followed by Japan in December, then France in July

1989, Australia in November 1989, and Canada in December 1989. Germany and the Netherlands waited until July 1995.[59] Sometimes the infected partners of those patients were included in the compensation packages – usually with a lesser amount of money, suggesting that sexual intercourse made the victim less innocent. Many of these countries have universal health care systems; compensation represented a symbolic acceptance of responsibility and an attempt to replace losses of employment income and to defray the costs of illness. It was a recognition of the nation's failure to protect its citizens from harm. People who contracted AIDS in other ways were not compensated.

In the United States, especially, the monetary needs of the sick are staggering because of inadequate medicare, expensive private health care, steep insurance premiums, and the fact that millions of people have no health insurance coverage at all. Money matters to Americans who are mortally ill. But the U.S. government has never offered compensation to people infected with AIDS by blood.[60]

In Canada, two delays in the management of AIDS later became relevant to hepatitis. First, Canada did not implement surrogate testing for AIDS. Surrogate testing was a means of using a blood test for other conditions which also tended to occur in people with AIDS although not exclusively. Instead, Canada waited until November 1985 to begin HIV screening, while some jurisdictions in the United States had been using surrogates since mid-1984 and distributing testing kits by March 1985.[61] Second, heat-treated concentrates for hemophiliacs were less dangerous than those that had not been treated with heat, but the best method for heating the factor concentrates was not established before May 1986. By then, wet heat was found to be more effective than dry heat, but Canada's stock of dry-heat-treated concentrate (prepared from paid donors) was not recalled until November 1986. Six hemophiliacs in British Columbia, five of them children, contracted HIV in this 1984–6 period while using dry-heat-treated concentrate. They were each awarded $1.55 million from Armour Pharmaceutical Company.[62]

Just like AIDS, hepatitis was transmitted by blood. Once blood banks began screening for AIDS (in the United States by May 1985, in Canada by November 1985), a parallel drop in the incidence of post-transfusion hepatitis took place, 90 per cent of which was hepatitis non-A non-B.[63] According to the only study done in Canada, detectable hepatitis followed 9 per cent of transfusions in 1985 – a rate similar to that of the United States. After controls for AIDS prevention were implemented, the hepatitis rate dropped to 2 per cent.[64] These figures implied that donors who were infected with HIV were also likely to be carriers of hepatitis non-A non-B.

Hepatitis research did not go away, but it proceeded slowly. The histories of hepatitis C list certain 'milestones,' stations of the cross, small skirmishes in winning a war.[65] The objective was to identify the virus that caused hepatitis non-A non-B, if it was a virus, and to invent a test for it. A long-term goal would be to find the cause and treatments for the unexplained chronic liver diseases. But the immediate goal was to identify the virus in people who had no symptoms at all so that they would not continue to contaminate the blood supply. Did anyone wonder what would happen when a host of symptomless people would be labelled as dangerously ill? That would be the most radical change in the concept of hepatitis in over 2500 years.

These 'milestones' in hepatitis C research can be reviewed quickly. In the mid-1970s, Daniel W. Bradley of the Centers for Disease Control succeeded in infecting chimpanzees with hepatitis non-A non-B from human blood.[66] He proved that it was an infectious disease according to Koch's postulates,[67] and his methods served as a model for AIDS scientists who infected chimps with HIV in 1984.[68] Bradley's work also allowed for clinical analysis of the course of the illness and its effects. Hepatitis non-A non-B had a long natural history: 60 per cent of the chimps were still sick one year after infection, and liver signs persisted for well over five years. The illness smouldered; however, symptoms were often absent and liver function was only mildly disturbed with elevation of the enzyme alanine aminotransferase (or ALT). Bradley postulated that the virus remained active in the host organism for life.

Bradley's chimps, together with other observations made in a European dialysis unit, implied that performing liver function tests on donated blood would serve as a useful 'surrogate' test for the elusive virus.[69] An elevation of ALT enzyme implied that the donor *might* have hepatitis and the blood should be discarded. A similar suggestion had been made as early as 1959.[70] But ALT is sensitive to many liver changes; for example, it would be elevated in blood donated after a night of carousing. With this method, it seemed that many uninfected units of blood would be thrown away, creating even bigger supply problems for blood bankers. The scientific fixation on viruses as specific causes for hepatitis was also instrumental in the repeated decisions not to use surrogate tests for preventing post-transfusion hepatitis. Like the Canadian blood bankers who waited for HIV tests, scientists preferred to use (and wait for) specific tests that would finally identify the hypothetical virus.[71]

By August 1981, Harvey J. Alter's team at the NIH proved that nearly 30 per cent of post-transfusion hepatitis could be prevented by surrogate testing with ALT.[72] Similar predictions were made about the accuracy of using core antigen of hepatitis B virus as a surrogate for the other hepatitis.[73] Further reports of the value of surrogate tests came during 1984; with promises of up to 60 per cent reduction in post-transfusion hepatitis with surrogate testing, they dared to invoke the spectre of cost-benefit analysis. One study showed that subtracting the costs of performing the test on all donor units from the costs of caring for people with hepatitis would result in a net saving of over 700 dollars for every case prevented.[74]

Blood banks 'agonized' over the decision;[75] some chose to heed the advice to use surrogates in the absence of randomized, controlled trials. Germany launched such testing as early as July 1984; the United States in March 1986. Those who waited came to regret it. The Canadian Red Cross was one of the latter; as late as December 1986, it considered and rejected the idea. Canadians thought that the risk was negligible in their country and they worried about supplies.

In 1987, a conference held in London, UK, invited scientists who were working on hepatitis non-A non-B to present their findings. Four groups were studying the molecular biology of the possible virus. They had a gloomy sense that little progress had been made; most new results were in the realm of clinical characteristics of the disease. Without a single, specific cause, some were sceptical that it was a distinct disease at all. Lacking evidence-based proof for the value of expensive surrogate tests, others contended that the optimum solution was to wait, hoping 'for a randomized controlled trial which never appeared.'[76] Yet no one dared to conduct a randomized study that would subject some patients to the risk of blood that had not been examined by surrogate tests.

In December 1987, two researchers rose to the occasion: S. Victor Feinman of Mount Sinai Hospital in Toronto and Morris A. Blajchman, director of the Hamilton Red Cross and a professor at McMaster University. They applied for funding to conduct a randomized, controlled study of the value of surrogate tests in preventing transfusion hepatitis on the Canadian population.[77] They argued that because Canada was not using the tests, the so-called 'untreated control group' was the norm in that country. About five thousand transfusions would be needed to demonstrate the advantages, if any, of surrogate tests. The results would take some time, but obtaining the funding took much longer. The Canadian Blood Committee funded care and supply of blood; it was not accustomed to funding research and the Red Cross officials were opposed to surrogate testing.[78] During the wait for funding, exciting events in the world of hepatitis research overtook this project in transfusion research.

Hepatitis C

Finally, the combined teams of Daniel Bradley, at the Centers for Disease Control in Atlanta, and of Michael Houghton, at Chiron Laboratories in Emeryville, California, announced that they had cloned the virus that caused hepatitis non-A non-B.[79] They published the results in April 1989, back to back with another article describing an assay to identify the virus.[80] This success followed a year of exciting announcements.[81] Again, the name of the disease changed, this time to hepatitis C. At first, the researchers had not known if they were looking for an RNA or a DNA virus; however, by extracting nucleic acid from vast amounts of plasma taken from infected chimps, they established that the hepatitis C virus is small, single-stranded RNA virus bound to a nucleocapsid with a glycoprotein envelope. How did they know they had the right virus?

Scientists were ready for the question. The Houghton team had to test their presumed virus against a mystery panel of serums – some were infected; some, not. The code was broken to show that all but one serum had been successfully identified, and the excited researchers popped corks. Another victory for industrial science, and we are grateful. Why was industry interested? At the end of the long, dark tunnel was a bright promise of returns from sales of a test kit that would be used on every unit of blood in every blood bank around the world – a test kit for which Chiron Laboratories would hold the patent. Commercial forces play a role in defining disease, as well as in finding cures.

This feat took place entirely within a tried-and-true paradigm, but it was difficult and in some ways 'unprecedented.' Harvey Alter explained the originality in his intriguing article 'Descartes before the Horse: I Clone therefore I Am': the hepatitis C virus (HCV) was cloned before it had been 'substantiated through tissue culures, microscopic observation, serologic identification, or genomic characterization.'[82] HCV is variable, with more than 100 different subtypes; it does not grow easily in cell culture. As of mid-2002, it had still not been characterized morphologically or biochemically.[83] Fourteen years after the so-called discovery of this virus, no one had determined its exact shape or composition, although attempts were ongoing.

Nevertheless, tests for HCV became available; by June 1990, they were applied in Canada.[84] The incidence of post-transfusion hepatitis dropped further from a residual 1.5 per cent to almost zero. 'You'll wonder where the yellow went,' quipped Harvey Alter in the year 2000, as he accepted an award for his role in the discovery.[85]

The conceptual precision of a name, a causative agent, and a blood test meant that research could focus on the carrier state and chronic forms of the disease. Efforts began and are still ongoing to determine the natural history of the disease.

During all this time, Blajchman and Feinman had been waiting to collect data for their randomized trial on the value of surrogate tests. Funding from a variety of sources was finally approved for their study by September 1989, after almost two years of delays spent on ironing out criticisms of method and protocol: critics had argued over the 'mechanism of informed consent,' although no one suggested that the study was unnecessary.[86] Everyone expected a test kit for hepatitis C to be available soon, and once the test was implemented by Canadian officials, the study could require many more patients enrolled to demonstrate a beneficial difference within an improved system. The team collected data from more than 4600 blood donations in Toronto, Hamilton, and Winnipeg from September 1989 through March 1990, when the HCV test was implemented, and they carried on until the spring of 1993 using the surrogate test in addition to the HCV tests. For each case, they had to wait six months for the post-transfusion hepatitis to manifest itself, or not. At first, hepatitis was identified by a rise in liver enzymes, and later, it could be confirmed by the new tests to show the presence of hepatitis C with seroconversion. The trial continued after the advent of the hepatitis C test in order to answer two questions: did surrogate testing offer additional protection to that provided by HCV testing and was the newly identified HC virus responsible for all the remaining post-transfusion hepatitis?

In April 1993, Blajchman and Feinman reported that the incidence of post-transfusion hepatitis had been declining even before they began the study due to methods designed to eliminate HIV: from the 9.5 per cent reported in 1985 to less than 1.5 per cent in 1989.[87] When their study was complete, surrogates offered no advantage over hepatitis C testing, but recipients of blood screened only by surrogate tests had 40 per cent fewer cases of hepatitis and 70 per cent fewer instances of hepatitis C conversion (from 2 per cent to zero).[88] In other words, Blajchman and Feinman proved that surrogate testing would have been an effective way to prevent post-transfusion hepatitis had it been used. They were surprised. The results were released quietly at a meeting with Red Cross officials on 2 September 1993 and were published in January 1995.

The Blajchman-Feinman study might appear to have been merely of historical interest, as its final report came after the more precise HCV screening was available. Yes, it was the randomized double-blind study that researchers had once thought impossible. But it was much more: it was pivotal to the legal inquiry that followed. Blajchman and Feinman posed a disturbing explanatory challenge to those who believe that we should always wait for randomized, controlled trials before acting. They also brought the history of medicine squarely into the arena of public debate by providing irrefutable evidence about who should have done what, and when. Lawyers loved it. This study of Canadians by Canadians proved that the Canadian delay had been a mistake.

Why was the Blajchman-Feinman study released quietly? Certainly, the Red Cross was not eager to publicize results that would make it vulnerable to civil liability. But retrospective demonization is anachronistic and fails to consider the context. The delay in publication of the Blajchman-Feinman study was typical of scientific publishing; it was rejected by a first journal and then subjected to a 'fairly smooth' peer-review process by the *Lancet*, which eventually accepted it.[89] Hepatitis had long been a well-known risk in the territory of transfusion, especially when its relative incidence was much higher. By 1993, media interest in transfusion-related AIDS was far greater than its interest in transfusion-related hepatitis (figure 3.2).[90] The discovery of the HC virus four years earlier had been big news for science. For the general public, however, the disease of hepatitis C barely existed. Things were about to change dramatically.

Hepatitis C and Horace Krever, or How the Law Constructs Disease

The safety of blood, like the safety of drugs, is the responsibility of the state and the provider. If blood makes someone sick, then compensation can be sought but not necessarily granted. In the United States, where private health care is expensive and blood products have long been bought and sold, injured recipients have appealed to the courts. But lawsuits brought by Americans against hospitals and blood banks for transfusion-associated hepatitis have met with little success. A probably incomplete survey of cases concerning transfusion-associated hepatitis

Figure 3.2 Media reports on transfused HIV and hepatitis, 1983–1993

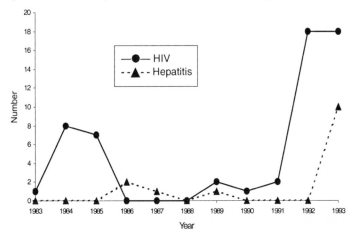

Source: Canadian BCA database. This chart was prepared by keyword searches combining 'HIV' or 'hepatitis' with the words 'tainted' or 'transfus/ion/ed.'

through the Quicklaw database produced eighteen actions, tried between 1951 and 1989, in fifteen U.S. states, and at three court levels. Only five found in favour of the blood recipient who had contracted hepatitis (in one case, it was the family of a deceased recipient): four were at the level of the supreme courts; one, at the appellate level. All five judgments were given with dissenting opinions, and new trials may not have been pursued.[91]

To the best of my knowledge, Canadians who contracted hepatitis, syphilis, or other infections from blood were never compensated as a group or as individuals until after the advent of AIDS. On the other hand, venereal infection as a form of assault has a long legal history in Canada and Britain with a stark reversal in attitude over the last century and a half. In 1878 and again in 1998, concealment of venereal infection to induce consent for sexual relations was presented as a form of fraud. But times change. The judgment went in favour of the defendant in 1878 and against in 1998.[92]

In October 1992, three officials of the French national transfusion service went to jail for criminal negligence in that nation's AIDS tragedy.[93] They were sentenced to prison terms of up to four years for failing to protect the blood supply with measures that had been successfully implemented elsewhere. The court found that they had been lax in weighing human cost against monetary cost in an actuarial fashion and in failing to imagine the harmful consequences of their deliberations. National pride had preceded this downfall, because the officials had preferred to wait for French science, rather than following American actions. The sensational story was carried by press services around the globe. It worried some researchers who, in sympathy with convicted scientist J.P. Allain, recalled past uncertainties and constraints on publicly funded agencies.[94] It meant that people could be guilty of causing a disease even as they were supposed to be aiming for prevention. It suggested that no one was immune to prosecution, anywhere.

The Canadian media and the general public became sensitized to the problem of hepatitis C by the Commission of Inquiry on the Blood System in Canada. Organized in autumn 1993 and chaired by the distinguished jurist Horace Krever, hearings were held in every province except Prince Edward Island during 1994 and 1995. Originally created to examine the response to HIV/AIDS, this inquiry not only alerted the country to the existence of another new disease, it caused an unprecedented 'epidemic' in reported cases of hepatitis.

As the Krever Inquiry proceeded, 'innocent' hepatitis patients in Canada protested the unfairness of compensation for post-transfusion AIDS and not for post-transfusion hepatitis. Those known to have been infected with hepatitis during the window of injudicious delay – between the American implementation of surrogate tests and the advent of hepatitis C screening – had an even greater claim to have been wronged. What happened in other countries influenced perceptions of what ought to have happened at home. Italy had been compensating those with liver disease since February 1992. In Ireland, a group of mothers who had been infected with HCV by blood products used to prevent Rh-disease in their future newborns (erythroblastosis foetalis) began demanding compensation that was eventually granted in 1995.[95] Lawyers, judges, reporters, bureaucrats, doctors, politicians, and the general public soon became experts on the various tests for protecting the blood supply and on the dates of their release or implementation at home and abroad.

By December 1995, Krever issued a notice of possible wrongdoing to ninety-five Canadians who had been involved with the administration of the blood supply or the health care system, including doctors, bureaucrats, pharmaceutical and Red Cross officials, high-ranking politicians, including provincial ministers of health and several premiers, and Her Majesty the Queen in right of provinces and territories. This action outraged some of the most powerful of these people, who tried to thwart Krever's investigation by launching a court challenge to his jurisdiction.[96] The commission now attracted international attention in a media feeding frenzy that was fuelled by memory of the prison terms handed to officials in France. At that moment, hepatitis C was receiving more media interest than HIV (compare figures 3.2 and 3.3).

During the Krever inquiry it emerged that the Canadian Blood Committee had destroyed papers and erased tapes in response to an Access to Information request from a journalist.[97] Two former Red Cross directors were paid their salaries – what seemed like huge sums of money – for their time given to preparation for their testimony and its delivery. Once again, politics entered medical literature: the British journal *Lancet* carried a photograph of Health Minister David Dingwall with the report of his abject apology in the House of Commons for the govern-

Figure 3.3 Media reports on transfused HIV and hepatitis, 1983–2002

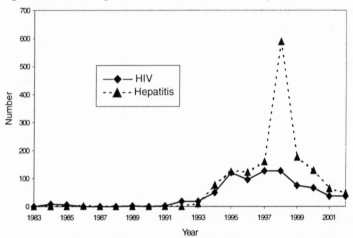

Source: Canadian BCA database. This chart was prepared by keyword searches combining 'HIV' or 'hepatitis' with the words 'tainted' or 'transfus/ion/ed.' Data for 2002 calculated based on information available at the time of writing.

ment lawyer's 'repugnant' accusation that Krever was conducting a 'witch hunt.'[98] Later, Health Minister Alan Rock was depicted in *Nature*.[99] The Supreme Court heard the case in May 1996 and dismissed the appeal the following month. Krever carried on. In late 1997, he released his report, amounting to over one thousand pages in three volumes. Not only does it contain well-documented histories of both AIDS and hepatitis in Canada and elsewhere, it is also a milestone in the history of the Red Cross and of all blood-borne diseases.[100]

The Blajchman-Feinman study contributed to the Krever inquiry. It had tried to answer the questions that no one else dared to explore, and its demonstration of the mistaken delay in surrogate testing justified the claims of victims. Citing Blajchman and Feinman, Krever concluded that 'The decision of the Red Cross not to implement anti-HBc and ALT testing of blood donations in Canada as surrogates for Non-A, Non-B hepatitis was not an acceptable one.'[101] Ironically, Morris Blajchman was moved to tears in reading his own statement to the Krever inquiry on the demands for scientific information placed on him and other blood scientists, the frustrating absence of research funding, and the steady pressure for more blood. At the hearings some witnesses contended that Blajchman and Feinman's research was unethical and should never have been done, yet, at least one of those witnesses had been a reviewer of the original grant, which had been given a *unanimously* high rating. That witness must have changed his mind about the ethics of the research some time between the granting process and the inquiry. The Blajchman-Feinman study, like those of Saul Krugman, has been retrospectively demonized.[102]

With others, Blajchman now claims that the field of transfusion medicine is shunned by residents, and his sense of frustration and betrayal persists.[103] He is not alone in these feelings.[104] Already disgraced by the negligence and apparent cupidity of its officials, the Canadian Red Cross lost its role as a player in transfusion medicine, and its legal and financial troubles are still not over.[105] Krever recommended changes in the management of the blood supply and called for a new blood collection agency.[106]

Krever also found that Canada's method of compensation (for AIDS but not for hepatitis) was 'unfair.'[107] To illustrate his point, he cited the story of a British family who had lost three hemophiliac sons. The family received compensation for the two boys who had died of AIDS, but nothing for the lad who died of hepatitis.[108] His report urged funds 'for compensating persons who suffer serious consequences as a result of the administration of blood components or blood products.'[109] Once accused of conducting a 'witch hunt,' Krever wrote eloquently of the problems of the tort system, which requires a finding of 'fault' in order to provide financial relief if not compensation; instead, he recommended a no-fault system for compensating blood-injured persons.[110] The conceptual tyranny of this aspect of our legal system is not unlike the tyranny of a diagnostic system that privileges specific disease entities when, sometimes, no diagnoses are to be found.[111]

In the final report, Krever did not name names, nor did he specify what he meant by 'serious consequences of the administration of blood.' For lack of a better definition, we rely on seroconversion, a blood test that reveals the presence of a virus. In August 1997, while waiting for the final report, aggrieved citizens who were infected with hepatitis C threatened a class action suit hoping to convince the government to compensate them without going to court.[112] The heightened awareness led many people to seek testing and created an unprecedented 'epidemic' of hepatitis C in Canada even as transfusion hepatitis waned (see figure 3.4 and contrast with figure 3.1).[113] It is not known how many of the reported cases were symptomatic. The trigger was not the discovery of the virus, nor the advent of screening tests, but the Krever inquiry itself. The disease now appeared to be contagious through a media vector.

On 27 March 1998, the federal government announced a $1.2 billion compensation package. Benefits were to be paid only to those people who should have been protected by surrogate tests for hepatitis had Canada implemented them.[114] An early cut-off date for eligibility could have been chosen, such as 1984 (when Germany implemented the tests), but the Canadian government chose 1986, when the United States had implemented the tests. People infected with HCV by blood prior to 1986 were not eligible for compensation. The reasoning was that HCV infection prior to the surrogate tests was an unavoidable accident, just as any hepatitis leaking through the system would be now. Public furor at this news escalated (plate 3.2): the amounts were considered too small and the cut-off date of 1986 was considered arbitrary.[115] Each province considered the matter separately. Ontario was quick to supplement the federal

Figure 3.4 Incidence and types of hepatitis reported in Canada

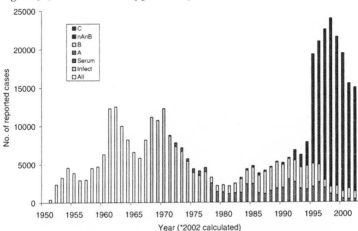

Source: Mosley, 1969; DBSTATS, 1968–74; CDWR 1974–79 CCDR 1994, 2002.*
Contrast this 'epidemic' with the decline of transfusion hepatitis in fig. 3.1.

offer and in June 2001 approved compensation for those
infected prior to 1986 who had been left out of the original
agreement.[116] Quebec and British Columbia soon followed suit.

During this period the number of Canadians who had
become infected with HIV or hepatitis was known to be around
1100 (at least 700 of whom were hemophiliacs).[117] But the numbers infected with hepatitis C, possibly with no symptoms, were
unknown but thought to be many more: estimates ranged from
17,000 to 240,000.[118] They were calculated on the number of
units of blood transfused (300,000 per year) and the incidence of
HCV in the donor pool (about 0.8 per cent). As many as 80,000
people were thought to be eligible for compensation from the
government; if the period of compensation were to be rolled
back to the early 1980s, then an additional 60,000 people would
have to be compensated.[119] These calculations assumed that all
recipients of blood would have survived their original illness.
At one point, the *Lancet* reported that 12,000 Canadians had

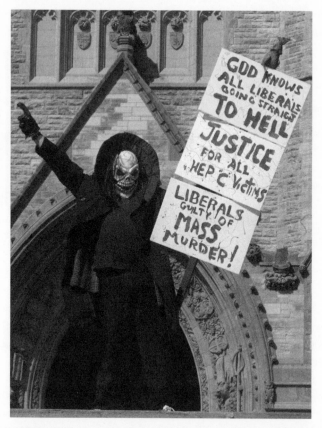

Plate 3.2 Death demonstrating ('Seeing Red,' *Kingston Whig-Standard*, 21 September 2000, 14).

already contracted hepatitis C from blood products '15% of whom are expected to die.'[120] I've got news for *Lancet*: all of them are expected to die some day, and all of us too. The difficulty with hepatitis C prognosis is this: it *can* kill you, making you and your family miserable while it does, but we don't know if it *will* kill you, or when. Was symptomless presence of HCV sufficient to warrant financial compensation? Would many people receive money only to remain healthy? Italy dealt with the matter by giving compensation to those who had demonstrable liver disease rather than seropositivity.[121]

The Natural History of Hepatitis C

The natural history of the disease was not understood. Several prospective and retrospective studies have tried to pin down the incidence and the outcome of HCV infection. Consensus conferences on the subject were held in Vienna in October 1995, in Bethesda in March 1997, and in Montreal in May 2001.[122] The Bethesda conference was hosted by the NIH, but it had commercial sponsorship from Amgen firm. In trying to establish all aspects of the natural history, the cost-benefit ratios were thought to be approximately $4000 saved for every case of HCV seropositivity found.[123] As a result, some hospitals conducted studies to notify those who were eligible for testing because of transfusions that they had received in the critical period and beyond. In these studies, more than half of those contacted had died, but a high proportion of living recipients had seroconverted to hepatitis C.[124]

The clinical news is sobering. Up to 80 per cent of people exposed to hepatitis C will go on to develop chronic infection. Of those, 10 per cent will have cirrhosis in ten years; the figure may be as high as 20 per cent after twenty years. A smaller but significant number will develop liver cancer. Four million people are estimated to be infected in the United States and around 170 million worldwide (or 3 per cent of the globe's population).[125] As of spring 2002, 8000 to 10,000 people die each year in the United States from complications of the infection. But these estimates are soft; not enough time has elapsed since the identification of the virus for the long-term prognosis to be established with confidence, and the life expectancy for those infected may increase or decrease from the figures we use now. For example, hepatitis C concentrates in saliva and transmission to dental workers is postulated but not established. Given the prevalence of the virus, a host of communication possibilities arise.[126]

But not all the news is bad. Of every hundred people infected with hepatitis C, eighty have no symptoms, and so far it is thought that only three will die because of it.[127] Vaccines have proved effective in chimps.[128] It appears that the vast majority of those infected will either recover completely or manage with stable illness. The U.S. incidence has declined from 240,000 cases per year in the early 1980s to 25,000 by 2001.[129] Treatments are still supportive, rather than curative; however, new drugs are coming, interferon is helpful, and up to half of the cases of hepatitis C resolve spontaneously, depending on the subtype of virus.[130] Infection combined with alcohol abuse has a poor prognosis. Indeed, alcohol itself remains a more frequent and more damaging cause of liver disease than HCV. Speaking in Montreal in 2001, Harvey Alter reported that 'a non-drinker with the virus has a better chance than a drinker without.'[131]

The genetic variation of HCV meant that researchers could undertake epidemiological studies to characterize the incidence, type, and route of HCV infection in their institution, region, or country.[132] For example, Prince Edward Island reported that half of cases involved drug users, 44 per cent of cases were the result of transfusions, and the remaining 5 per cent were unexplained.[133] A study of ninety-two patients from northern Alberta found that 'lifestyle' was a more reliable predictor of HC infection than was transfusion.[134] The regional findings by subtype could eventually give a molecular history of the ecology of the virus.[135]

The natural history of the disease has been investigated in a number of retrospective studies of preserved blood. Tests done recently on serum drawn in 1945 from more than 8000 U.S. troops revealed that seventeen of the soldiers had been carriers of HCV. Seven were dead, one of whom had succumbed to liver disease two full decades after his blood was drawn. Ten of the seventeen were still alive and well forty-five years later.[136]

Other indications of the natural history of hepatitis C can be derived from Canada's experience with the compensation package. To date, fewer Canadians came forward for compensation than had been predicted. Four and a half years after the compensation package was announced, only $200 million, or one-sixth, of the full $1.2 billion package had been paid out. Disbursements included $52 million to lawyers and $9 million for administration; 4,946 people had been awarded just over $40,000 each, considerably less than anticipated.[137] The government rejected the claims of more than 800 people; sometimes the infection fell outside the period of compensation, or the claimant admitted to other possible sources of infection, such as the 'adolescent indiscretion' of IV drug use.[138] In one 'look-back' study, only a third of those contacted actually responded; 32 per cent of the respondents had not known that they had been transfused, although they were grateful for information and the opportunity to be tested.[139] Similar results of a 'look-back' study at the Hospital for Sick Children in Toronto led researchers to suggest that children may be better able to resist infection when transfused with the virus.[140]

The original predictions of how many people would be eligible for compensation seemed to have ignored the well-known fact that roughly 50 per cent of all people receiving blood transfusions would be dead within five years – not because of the transfusion, but because of the underlying condition that had necessitated it.[141] In other words, the natural history of hepatitis C depends not only on the route of infection, but also on the presence of other diseases.

Conclusion

In the wake of the legal and political turmoil, and conditioned by a cultural posture often referred to as 'victim-itis,' hepatitis C changed again by dividing into two diseases. At the moment, they bear the same name and the distinctions may be difficult to see, but the four disease theories, discussed in chapter 1, will help to sharpen them.

The first disease is usually symptomless and identified only by a positive blood test, which makes the sufferer eligible for money from the Canadian government. Mr R. was right: a few thousand dollars is not much money for a life, were it intended to be that. Instead, the compensation is a symbolic admission of responsibility. An as-yet-unknown percentage of these people will go on to develop severe liver disease, which will then resemble (but not be) the second disease. Some – half or more – will stay healthy with respect to their livers; most will die of something else. But they will all die of something, sometime. This virtually asymptomatic illness of HCV seropositivity has been 'out there' for at least fifty years, certainly as long as doctors have known of the mysterious conditions of chronic active hepatitis and cryptogenic cirrhosis. But the disease itself and its epidemic are new.

This symptom-free hepatitis C is a disease that conforms to the ontological theory (as presented in chapter 1). It is caused by an invading organism and also by other factors *external* to the patient: by the scientific discoveries; by the Krever inquiry; by journalists, politicians, lawyers, and jurists; and by the compensation packages. Yet, the number of people who are actually sick with liver symptoms may not be significantly different from what it was in the past. We have good reason to believe it is much lower (compare figures 3.1 and 3.4).

The second hepatitis C disease is a serious, chronic liver inflammation with many symptoms that may or may not be connected to blood contamination and for which no compensation is paid. It is carried by about 0.05 per cent of completely healthy Canadians who have never had a transfusion and whose blood, should they donate, will be thrown away. Considerable geographic differences in incidence have been documented.[142] The progress of this disease can also lead to more serious conditions, such as cirrhosis or cancer. Today most hepatitis C in Canada is of this second type. Only a small percentage resulted from blood transfusions, while approximately 70 per cent of cases are associated with intravenous drug use.[143] In this category, the proportion of transfusion-induced cases will continue to wane because new cases caused by blood have not appeared since 1995. This type of hepatitis C seems to be related to behaviour: the use of street drugs; having sex with a street-drug user; living with a street-drug user; being jailed; living with someone who was jailed; and participating in a Japanese form of frequent, violent heterosexual sex.[144] In at least 5 per cent of cases, the route of infection is unknown. Only a few scientists and even fewer journalists seem to be interested in the causes or treatment for the second type of hepatitis C.

This second, symptom-rich type of hepatitis C conforms to the *physiological* theory of disease (as discussed in chapter 1). It is caused by a virus, yes, but it is also the result of the character or behaviour of the patient. It matters who the patient is and what she does, and she can be blamed for her troubles. I submit that this condition is the 'guilty' variety of hepatitis C. It is less worthy of consideration than the first, 'innocent,' type in terms of research for treatment and prevention, and in terms of journalistic interest. Why? Perhaps because little money is to be made by lawyers or pharmaceutical companies or journalists from attention to the afflicted, and, especially, because we *tolerate* (even if we do not approve of) negative attitudes toward the sufferers. The distinction between the two types of hepatitis C is reinforced, not only by the differing routes of infection, but also by compensation packages, which lend dignity to those with the 'innocent' type and focus blame on others with the 'guilty' type.

To illustrate this dichotomy, consider the interesting accusation made in March 2002 by Pamela Anderson, the beautiful

Canadian actress of the famously artificial breasts. She alleged that her ex-husband gave her hepatitis C from a shared tattoo needle. The same *Globe and Mail* article reported that the disease could also be spread by sex.[145] Since the couple had two children, they must have had unprotected sex at least twice. How can Anderson be confident that her contamination came from the tattoo needle and not from her cosmetic surgery or from making love? Did she select the route of infection most likely to highlight her innocence? Was she attempting to leap from the guilty form of hepatitis C to the innocent, by emphasizing the culpability of someone else?

Why are people who have non-transfusion HCV ineligible for compensation? On the surface, we say it is because their sickness cannot be the fault of the public trust. But this distinction about trust represents yet another manifestation of the power of the medical model, the *organismic* theory. We resist thinking of any disease in the collective. Disease must affect individuals.

Let me be clear: I am not trying to suggest that all sufferers should be compensated. More is the wonder to me that, in a country with relatively free health care, any group of people, with any disease, should be compensated in dollars at all, especially when the process includes some sufferers and not all. Ostensibly, compensation is to replace lost income and costs of illness; but all patients will suffer the same financial burden. Money acknowledges responsibility, but it will not cure the disease; nor will it right the wrong. Even the recipients of compensation will agree with that.

Let us now set aside that dominant medical model, the organismic theory, and consider another hypothesis: that the second, more frequent, 'guilty' form of hepatitis C resides in and is tolerated by the entire population. Geographic and social factors influence the distribution of hepatitis C. Prisoners who contract the disease in jail are at the mercy of the public, which has failed to protect them from the harm of incarceration: shared razors, drug use, dirty tattoo needles, rape, and sexually transmitted infections.[146] People who abuse substances, either in prison or on the street, have also been let down by the public in two ways: first, for its failure to control drug crime; second, for its failure to provide a balanced living environment that would allay the original impulse to use. Our whole society could see itself as afflicted collectively and uncomplainingly by this guilty form of hepatitis C. By extrapolation, society might even see itself as a cause. A population view would have hepatitis C as tolerable and continuous and its treatment and prevention would be aimed at social problems. But the population view is not how disease concepts work. The sick are weak and rarely in a position to bring their plight to public attention; it is easy to blame the sufferers themselves for being inadequate, pitiable, and criminal. These prejudicial attitudes take on an exaggerated allure of logic through the disease theories that we use to construct medical problems: one has power, the other does not. The organismic theory (medical model) governs the construct. Diseases must occur in individuals, not in collectives. Society can be let off the hook.

And finally, what does hepatitis have to do with love? I am far from being the first to make a connection: back in 1759, Jerome David Gaub warned that jaundice was one of the serious physical ailments caused by love.[147] In our own time, love contributes to the duality of hepatitis C. AIDS provides the pattern, just as syphilis did in the past: they are diseases emblematic of their transmission to and from lovers.[148] Those who contracted AIDS from sexual partners are not compensated – unless the partner originally got it from blood, in which case the compensation is less for the sexual partner than for the blood recipient.[149]

Hepatitis C occurs among those who live with the inadequate, pitiable criminals, described above, sharing their tattoo needles, their beds, and their toothbrushes only to become infected too. They are lovers. Lovers who unwisely chose the tainted, and somehow become tainted themselves.

But the sexual transmission of hepatitis C is merely presumed, not proven. The tiny handful of scientists who work on this 'guilty,' nontransfusion-related hepatitis C seem to be preoccupied – if not obsessed – with the possibility that it is spread by sex. The chimpanzee investigations did not clarify the sexual transmission, and now we look to epidemiological surveys of humans rather than experiments on animals. So far, the reports reveal suspicion rather than confirmation of sexual transmission; they speak of significant negatives, slender correlations, and controversy.[150] Some studies suggest that sexual transmission is 'absent' or negligible;[151] others report rates as high as 27 per cent.[152] Nevertheless, sexual causes and sexual precautions curiously dominate current recommendations. In the *Canada Communicable Diseases Report*, hepatitis C is now grouped with the diseases spread by blood or sex, in between gonorrhea and syphilis; hepatitis B and A are dealt with elsewhere.[153] Similarly, the U.S. Centers for Disease Control (CDC) shows that the proportion of hepatitis C owing to sexual transmission rose as the transfusion causes declined – blood and sex.[154] Admitting that sexual spread is 'rare,' the CDC urges condom use.[155] The search for sexual transmission is as much for exoneration of the rest of us, as it is for a cause. 'Oh! She got it from sex. Sex with an infected loser. No wonder. Serves her right. Not my fault.' A lover is cause and embodiment of her disease.

Further implicating love as a cause of this disease is the origin of the tainted blood itself. Here I hearken back to the observation made in chapter 2, that our mistrust of lovers is not limited to our ambivalence over sex. No one in Canada has ever been paid for regularly donating blood; since the late 1970s, the practice has declined in the United States. A blood donation was thought to be a charitable offering from volunteers. It used to be called the 'Gift of Life.' Following AIDS, giving declined and selfishness rose: numbers of blood donations dropped. We have also seen the advent of private blood banks, which allow the apprehensive wealthy to store units of their own blood against future operations or potential accidents that might occur conveniently close to their freezer.

We must never forget that the 'tainted' people who donated their 'tainted' blood did it to help, out of charity, as an act of love. The recipients of the well-intended gift are cast as the innocent aggrieved, wounded by an act of love. Those who cared enough to donate are cast as their guilty assailants. And when the guilty givers fall ill, they will suffer in exactly the same ways as their innocent-victim recipients. But they will do so unremunerated and unrecognized, just as they shared their blood.

Old or new, diseases are ideas.

Appendix:
'The Disease Game'
Homework Assignment

1. Using the guide to disease concepts in table 1.4, read three of the following four passages and determine what theory(ies) of disease influenced those who wrote these passages. Then give your reasons. Point form is OK.
2. Write your name in the space provided at the top of this page.
3. Hand in your homework for marking at the lecture tomorrow.

REMEMBER: There are no right or wrong answers; only good or bad explanations.

PRIZES on Thursday!

(For details of 'What Happened,' see the end of the Appendix.)

1 Gout attacks such old men as, after passing the best part of their life in ease and comfort, indulging freely in high living, wine, and other generous drinks, at length from inactivity, the usual attendant of advanced life, have left off altogether the bodily exercises of their youth ... The victim goes to bed and sleeps in good health. About two o'clock in the morning he is awakened by a severe pain in the great toe ... For humble individuals like myself, there is one poor comfort ... gout, unlike any other disease, kills more rich men than poor, more wise

men than simple ... Gout will take up its quarters even in a young subject and its empire will be no government, but a tyranny. (Thomas Sydenham, *Tractatus de Podagra et de Hydrope*, 1683)

2 A rare brain disease that has killed 10 people is probably linked to 'mad cow disease,' the [British] government said yesterday ... [T]here is evidence to connect a new strain of Creuzfeldt-Jakob disease [CJD] in humans with bovine spongiform encephalopathy, known as mad cow disease. ... The incurable disease [in humans] causes holes in the brain tissue, disabling and finally killing victims ... [T]he government still believes British milk and beef are safe ... [officials] said earlier there was no evidence that the disease could jump between species and infect people, although it is believed that mad cow disease jumped from sheep to cattle. After a rise of [CJD] among young people – and a rise in the general population from 18 cases in 1990 to 56 cases in 1994 – the government set up a surveillance unit ... Researchers ... report that 10 [CJD] deaths were likely linked to a new strain of the disease ... the average age of the 10 victims was 27.5 years compared to 63 years in previous cases of the disease. ('Deaths May Be Linked to Diseased Beef,' *Kingston Whig-Standard*, 21 March 1996, 8)

3 I do not believe that the '*Sacred Disease*' is any more divine or sacred than any other disease but, on the contrary, has specific characteristics and a definite cause. ... the brain is the seat of this disease ... Should ... the passage of phlegm ... be blocked, the discharge enters the blood-vessels ... [T]he patient loses his voice and his wits. The hands become powerless and move convulsively ... Divergence of the eyes takes place ... froth ... appears at the lips. Patients who suffer from this disease have a premonitory indication of an attack. (Hippocrates, 'The Sacred Disease,' 5th century BC)

4 How indeed could the body develop a new malady, a late born disease? ... For there cannot be a new disease without a cause, introducing into the world, contrary to natural law, a coming-to-be from not-being ... For it is the things that sustain life which also cause sickness. There are no special seeds of disease ... if something previously non-existent has come to be ... the cause of this is the structure of our bodies, which varies from time to time in the combination of its elements. (Plutarch, *Table Talk, Moralia*, 1st to 2nd century AD)

What Happened?

Thirty-five members of the audience completed the assignment. The grand prize (a helium-filled, heart-shaped balloon and a box of chocolate truffles) went to Lynn Kennedy. The prize for second place (two helium-filled, heart-shaped balloons) was shared by Mark Eaton and a woman whose name I do not have. The entire audience was rewarded with a large basket of Hershey's chocolate kisses.

Notes

Chapter 1: The Disease Game

1 Robert Aronowitz, *Making Sense of Illness: Science, Society, and Disease* (Cambridge: Cambridge University Press, 1998); Georges Canguilhem, *On the Normal and the Pathological*, trans. Carolyn R. Fawcett and Robert S. Cohen (New York: Zone Books, 1989); Arthur L. Caplan, H. Tristram Englehardt Jr, and James McCartney, eds, *Concepts of Health and Disease: Interdisciplinary Perspectives* (Reading, MA: Addison-Wesley, 1981); Ludwik Fleck, *Genesis and Development of a Scientific Fact* (Chicago: University of Chicago Press, 1979); Michel Foucault, *Naissance de la clinique: une archéologie du regard médical* (Paris: Presses Universitaires de France, 1963); Mirko D. Grmek, 'Le concept de maladie,' in *La vie, les maladies, et l'histoire*, ed. Louise L. Lambrichs (Paris: Seuil, 2001), 21–8; Mirko D. Grmek, 'Le concept de maladie,' in *Histoire de la pensée médicale en Occident*, ed. Mirko D. Grmek and Bernardino Fantini, vol. 1: *Antiquité et moyen âge* (Paris: Seuil, 1995), 211–26, and vol. 2: *De la Renaissance aux Lumières* (Paris: Seuil, 1997), 157–76; Robert Hudson, *Disease and Its Control: The Shaping of Modern Thought* (Westport, CT: Greenwood, 1980); Lester S. King, *Medical Thinking: A Historical Preface* (Princeton, NJ: Princeton University Press, 1982); Guenter B. Risse, 'Health and Disease: History of the Concepts,' in *Encyclopedia of Bioethics*, 4 vols, ed. Warren T. Reich (New York: Free Press, 1978), 2: 579–85; Charles E. Rosenberg, ed., *Explaining Epidemics and Other*

Studies in the History of Medicine (Cambridge: Cambridge University Press, 1992); Charles E. Rosenberg and Janet L. Golden, eds, *Framing Disease: Studies in Cultural History* (New Brunswick, NJ: Rutgers University Press, 1992); Oswei Temkin, 'The Scientific Approach to Disease: Specific Entity or Individual Sickness,' in *The Double Face of Janus* (Baltimore and London: Johns Hopkins University Press, [1963] 1977), 441–55.

2 Mirko D. Grmek, 'Un concept nouveau: la pathocénose,' in *La vie, les maladies, et l'histoire*, ed. Lambrichs, 29–33.

3 Guenter B. Risse, 'Epidemics and Medicine: The Influence of Disease on Medical Thought and Practice,' *Bulletin of the History of Medicine* 53 (1979): 505–19; Lloyd G. Stevenson, 'Exemplary Disease: The Typhoid Pattern,' *Journal of the History of Medicine* 37 (1982): 159–82.

4 For disease concepts in the early modern period, the writings of Lester S. King are particularly helpful. See Lester S. King, *Medical Thinking: The Medical World of the Eighteenth Century* (Chicago: University of Chicago Press, 1958), 193–226; *The Road to Medical Enlightenment* (London and New York: Macdonald and American Elsevier, 1970). See also Grmek, *Histoire de la pensée médicale en Occident*, 2: 157–76; William F. Bynum and Roy Porter, eds, *Medicine and the Five Senses* (Cambridge: Cambridge University Press, 1993).

5 Published in successive editions since 1952 by the American Psychiatric Association, the current edition is the *Diagnostic and Statistical Manual (DSM)-IV* (Washington: American Psychiatric Association, 1994).

6 Charles E. Rosenberg, 'Introduction: Framing Disease: Illness, Society, and History,' in *Framing Disease*, ed. Rosenberg and Golden, xiii–xxvi, esp. xiii–xiv.

7 Histories of syphilis abound; the following are interesting examples: Fleck, *Genesis and Development of a Scientific Fact*; Claude Quétel, *History of Syphilis*, trans. Judith Braddock and Brian Pike (Cambridge: Polity, 1990); Theodor Rosebury, *Microbes and Morals: The Strange Story of Venereal Disease* (New York: Viking, 1971).

8 Mirko D. Grmek, *History of AIDS: Emergence and Origin of a Modern Pandemic*, trans. Russell C. Maulitz and Jacalyn Duffin (Princeton: Princeton University Press, 1990), 32–3.

9 On the role of the law in disease construction, see Andrew Malleson, *Whiplash and Other Useful Illnesses* (Montreal and Kingston: McGill-Queen's University Press, 2002); Janet A. Tighe, 'The Legal Art of Psychiatric Diagnosis: Searching for Reliability,' in *Framing Disease*, ed. Rosenberg and Golden, 206–28.

10 Hippocrates, *Hippocrates with an English Translation*, trans. W.H.S. Jones, Vol. 2 Loeb Classical Library (Cambridge, MA: Harvard University Press, [1923] 1998), 139–83, esp. 159–63.

11 K. Codell Carter, *The Rise of Causal Concepts of Disease: Case Histories* (Aldershot: Ashgate, 2003).

12 Fred Rosner, 'Hemophilia in Classic Rabbinic Texts,' *Journal of the History of Medicine and Allied Sciences* 49 (1994): 240–50.

13 Theodore H. Spaet, 'Platelets: The Bood Dust,' in *Blood Pure and Eloquent: A Story of Discovery, of People, and of Ideas*, ed. Maxwell M. Wintrobe (New York: McGraw Hill, 1980), 548–71; Oscar D. Ratnoff, 'Why Do People Bleed?' in *Blood Pure and Eloquent*, ed. Wintrobe, 600–57.

14 Herbert Weiner, 'From Simplicity to Complexity (1950–1990): The Case of Peptic Ulceration – Part I. Human Studies,' and 'Part II. Animal Studies,' *Psychosomatic Medicine* 53 (1991): 491–516 and 467–90.

15 Dale C. Smith, 'Appendicitis, Appendectomy, and the Surgeon,' *Bulletin of the History of Medicine* 70 (1996), 414–41; Jacalyn Duffin, 'The Great Canadian Peritonitis Debate, 1844–47,' *Histoire sociale/ Social History* 19 (1987): 407–24.

16 Magdelena Biernacka, 'History of Visceroptosis,' unpublished paper read at the annual meeting of the Royal College of Physicians and Surgeons of Canada, Halifax, 1996; Sandra W. Moss, 'Floating Kidneys,' in *Clio in the Clinic*, ed. Jacalyn Duffin (Oxford University Press and University of Toronto Press, 2005).

17 On the history and impact of Prozac, see Peter D. Kramer, *Listening to Prozac: A Psychiatrist Explores Antidepressant Drugs and the Remaking of Self* (New York: Penguin, 1993).

18 Elaine S. Berman, '"Too Little Bone": The Medicalization of Osteoporosis,' *Journal of Women's Health and Law* 1, no. 3 (2000): 257–77.

19 For example, see the full-page, colour advertisement for Pfizer's Viagra, featuring Senator Robert Dole, who reminds readers that 'It

takes Courage to ask your doctor about E.D.' *New York Times*, 20 April 1999, F6. Since the delivery of the Goodman lectures I have been besieged by spam e-mail from two disease-constructing, market-driven sources: one, Kandace Delorme (nllctmc@msn.com), notifying me of free 'gen*ric V*agra' and the other, 'mdBriefCase' (gcook1@mdbriefcase.com), asking, 'Are you screening for ED?' and supplying information that 82 per cent of Canadian men expect their doctors to ask after their sexual health. The latter acknowledges that it is part of a 'program supported by an unrestricted educational grant from Pfizer Canada Inc.'

20 Roy Moynihan, 'The Making of a Disease: Female Sexual Dysfunction,' *British Medical Journal* 326 (2003): 45–7.

21 On the history of CFS and other similar conditions, see Aronowitz, *Making Sense of Illness*, 19–38; Gary Holmes (and fifteen other authors), 'Chronic Fatigue Syndrome: A Working Case Definition,' *Annals of Internal Medicine* 108 (1988): 387–9; Hillary Johnson, *Osler's Web: Inside the Labyrinth of the Chronic Fatigue Syndrome* (New York: Penguin, 1996); Evelyn Kim, 'A Brief History of Chronic Fatigue Syndrome,' *JAMA* 272 (1994): 1070–1; Edward Shorter, *From Paralysis to Fatigue: A History of Psychosomatic Illness in the Modern Era* (New York and Toronto: The Free Press, 1992), 295–323; Terra Ziporyn, *Nameless Diseases* (New Brunswick, NJ: Rutgers University Press, 1992), 106–7, 117–18.

22 A synthetic history of medical semiology has yet to be written. Good accounts can be found for certain specific eras. For specific eras, see the sources in the reference notes immediately following.

23 Paul Potter, 'Some Principles of Hippocratic Nosology,' in *La maladie et les maladies dans la Collection Hippocratique; 6e Colloque International Hippocratique, 1987*, ed. Paul Potter, Gilles Maloney, and Jacques Desautels (Quebec: Éditions du Sphinx, 1990), 237–53; Paul Potter, *A Short Handbook of Hippocratic Medicine* (Quebec: Éditions du Sphinx, 1988), esp. 47–8.

24 Antoinette Stettler, 'Zeichen lesen und Zeichen deuten: zur Geschichte der medizinischen Semiotick,' *Gesnerus* 44 (1987), 33–54. On medieval diagnostics see Ortrun Riha, 'Subjektivität und Objektivität, Semiotik und Diagnostik. Eine Annäherung an der mittelalterlichen Krankheitsbegriff,' *Sudhoff's Archiv: Zeitschrift für*

Wissenschaftsgeschichte 80 (1996), 129–49; Faith Wallis, 'The Experience of the Book: Manuscripts, Texts, and the Role of Epistemology in Early Medieval Medicine,' in *Knowledge and the Scholarly Medical Traditions*, ed. Don Bates (Cambridge: Cambridge University Press, 1995), 101–26; Faith Wallis, 'Inventing Diagnosis: Theophilus's "De Urinis" in the Classroom,' *Dynamis* 20 (2000): 31–73; Faith Wallis, 'Signs and Senses: Diagnosis and Prognosis in Early Medieval Pulse and Urine Texts,' *Social History of Medicine* 13 (2000): 265–78. On early modern and Enlightenment semiology, see King, *Road to Medical Enlightenment*, 113–33; King, *Medical Thinking*, 73–104, 110–23; King, *Medical World of the Eighteenth Century*, 193–226; Ian Maclean, *Logic, Signs and Nature in the Renaissance: The Case of Learned Medicine* (Cambridge: Cambridge University Press, 2002); Brian K. Nance, 'Determining the Patient's Temperament: An Excursion into Seventeenth-Century Medical Semeiology,' *Bulletin of the History of Medicine* (1993): 417–38.

25 For the nineteenth-century advent of anatomoclinical medicine, see Michel Foucault, *Naissance de la clinique* (Paris: Presses Universitaires de France, 1963); Kenneth D. Keele, *The Evolution of Clinical Methods in Medicine* (Springfield, IL: Charles C. Thomas, 1963).

26 For the twentieth-century rise in medical technology, see Audrey B. Davis, *Medicine and Its Technology. An Introduction to the History of Medical Instrumentation* (Westport, CT, and London: Greenwood, 1981); Joel D. Howell, *Technology in the Hospital: Transforming Patient Care in the Early Twentieth Century* (Baltimore: Johns Hopkins University, 1995); Bettyann Kevles, *Naked to the Bone: Medical Imaging in the Twentieth Century* (New Brunswick, NJ: Rutgers University Press, 1997); Stanley Joel Reiser, *Medicine and the Reign of Technology* (Cambridge and New York: Cambridge University Press, 1979).

27 For recent criticism of the emphasis on medical technology, see Dorothy Nelkin and Laurence Tancredi, *Dangerous Diagnostics: The Social Power of Biological Information* (Chicago: University of Chicago Press, 1994); Neil Postman, *Technopoly: The Surrender of Culture to Technology* (New York: Vintage Books, 1993), 92–106; David Rothman, *Strangers at the Bedside* (New York: Basic Books, 1991); Edward Tenner, *Why Things Bite Back: Technology and the Revenge of Unintended Consequences* (New York: Alfred A. Knopf, 1996), 26–70.

28 On this problem, see Ziporyn, *Nameless Diseases*, 106–7, 118–19. See also Charles E. Rosenberg, 'The Tyranny of Diagnosis: Specific Entities and Individual Experience,' *Milbank Quarterly* 80 (2002): 237–60.

29 'Declare the past, diagnose the patient, foretell the future; practise these acts. As to diseases, make a habit of two things – to help, or at least to do no harm. *The art has three factors, the diseases, the patient, the physician.* The physician is the servant of the art. The patient must cooperate with the physician in combatting the disease.' Hippocrates, 'Epidemics I,' in *Hippocrates with an English Translation*, 147–211, esp. 165 (my emphasis). See also Danielle Gourevitch, *Le triangle hippocratique dans le monde gréco-romain: le malade, sa maladie et son médecin* (Rome: École française de Rome, 1984).

30 I explored the heuristic possibilities of this thought experiment in a short work of fiction, 'Grand Rounds: Osteodensosis,' *CMAJ* 165 (2001): 1609–11.

31 Charles Singer, 'The Visions of Hildegard of Bingen,' in *From Magic to Science: Essays on the Scientific Twilight* (New York: Dover, [1917] 1958), 199–240. See Norman Cousins, 'The Anatomy of an Illness (as Perceived by the Patient),' *New England Journal of Medicine* 295 (1976): 1458–63. This essay became the basis for a book of the same title. For a short review of this literature, see Jacalyn Duffin, 'Sick Doctors: Bayle and Laennec on Their Own Phthisis,' *Journal of the History of Medicine* 43 (1988): 165–82, esp. 165–6n.

32 See for example, John Z. Ayanian and Arnold M. Epstein. 'Differences in the Use of Procedures between Women and Men Hospitalized for Coronary Heart Disease.' *New England Journal of Medicine and Philosophy* 325 (1991), 221–5.

33 Annemarie Mol, *the body multiple: ontology in medical practice* (Durham, NC: Duke University Press, 2002).

34 See especially the articles in a special issue devoted to 'Concepts of Health and Disease,' *Journal of Medicine and Philosophy* 1, no. 3 (1976). See also W. Miller Brown, 'On Defining "Disease,"' *Journal of Medicine and Philosophy* 10 (1985): 311–28; Caplan et al., eds, *Concepts of Health and Disease*; Eric Cassell, 'Ideas in Conflict: The Rise and Fall (and Rise and Fall) of New Views of Disease,' *Daedalus* 115 (spring 1986): 19–41; George L. Engel, 'A Unified Concept of Health and Disease,' *Perspectives in Biology and Medicine* 3 (1960): 459–85;

Harold Merskey, 'Variable Meanings for the Definition of Disease,' *Journal of Medicine and Philosophy* 11 (1986): 215–32; Walter Riese, *The Conception of Disease, Its History, Its Versions and Its Nature* (New York, 1953).

35 For more on disease theories, see Hudson, *Disease and Its Control*; Risse, 'Health and Disease: History of the Concepts.'

36 On the two causal theories, see Temkin, 'Scientific Approach to Disease.' See also Charles E. Rosenberg, 'What Is Disease? In Memory of Oswei Temkin,' *Bulletin of the History of Medicine* 77 (2003): 491–505.

37 On the late nineteenth-century rise of causal theories, see especially Carter, *The Rise of Causal Concepts*.

38 On the nonorganismic theory, see George L. Engel, 'The Need for a New Medical Model: A Challenge for Biomedicine,' in *Concepts of Health and Disease*, ed. Caplan et al., 589–607; Risse, 'Health and Disease: History of the Concepts,' esp. 584–5; Geoffrey Rose, 'Sick Individuals and Sick Populations,' *International Journal of Epidemiology* 14 (1985): 32–8.

39 Robert A. Aronowitz, *Making Sense of Illness*, 187–9; Wulf Schiefenhovel, 'Perception, Expression, and Social Function of Pain: A Human Ethological View,' *Science in Context* 8 (1995): 31–46.

40 Grmek, *History of AIDS*, 99–109.

41 See for example, Aronowitz, *Making Sense of Illness*, 57–83; Paul Atkinson, *The Clinical Experience: The Construction and Reconstruction of Medical Reality* (Westmead, UK: Gower, 1981); Michel Bonduelle, Toby Gelfand, and Christopher G. Goetz, *Charcot: Constructing Neurology* (New York: Oxford University Press, 1995); Karl Figlio, 'Chlorosis and Chronic Disease in Nineteenth-Century Britain: The Social Construction of Somatic Illness in Capitalist Society,' *Social History* 3 (1978): 167–97; Peter Wright and Andrew Treacher, eds, *The Problem of Medical Knowledge: Examining the Social Construction of Medicine* (Edinburgh: Edinburgh University Press, 1982).

42 For examples of this critical approach as applied to a wide variety of topics, see Joan Jacobs Brumberg, *Fasting Girls: The Emergence of Anorexia Nervosa as a Modern Disease* (Cambridge, MA: Harvard University Press, 1988); André Cellard, *Histoire de la folie au Québec de 1600 à 1850: le désordre* (Montreal: Boreal, 1991); Georgina Feld-

berg, *Disease and Class: Tuberculosis and the Shaping of Modern North American Society* (New Brunswick, NJ: Rutgers University Press, 1995); Sander L. Gilman, *Difference and Pathology: Stereotypes of Sexuality, Race, and Madness* (Ithaca, NY: Cornell University Press, 1985); Stephen J. Kunitz, *Disease and Social Diversity: The European Impact on the Health of Non-Europeans* (New York: Oxford University Press, 1994); Andrew T. Scull, *The Most Solitary of Afflictions: Madness and Society in Britain, 1700–1900* (New Haven and London: Yale University Press, 1993).

43 Susan Sontag, *Illness as Metaphor* (New York: Farrar, Strauss, and Giroux, 1977).

44 See for example, Ian Hacking, *Rewriting the Soul: Multiple Personality and the Sciences of Memory* (Princeton, NJ: Princeton University Press, 1995), esp. 8–20; Allan Young, *The Harmony of Illusions: Inventing Post-Traumatic Stress Disorder* (Princeton, NJ: Princeton University Press, 1995), 5–10.

45 Rosenberg, 'Introduction: Framing Disease'; Roy Porter and G.S. Rousseau, *Gout: The Patrician Malady* (New Haven and London: Yale University Press, 1998), 1.

46 Mirko D. Grmek, 'Le concept de maladie émergente,' *History and Philosophy of the Life Sciences* 15 (1993): 281–96.

47 David Harley, 'Rhetoric and the Social Construction of Sickness and Healing,' *Social History of Medicine* 12 (1999): 407–35; Mol, *the body multiple*, 27, 152; Adrian Wilson, 'On the History of Disease-Concepts: The Case of Pleurisy,' *History of Science* 38 (2000): 271–319.

48 Bert Hansen, 'American Physicians' "Discovery" of Homosexuals, 1880–1900: A New Diagnosis in a Changing Society,' in *Framing Disease*, ed. Rosenberg and Golden, 104–33.

49 See the essays collected by H. Tristram Englehardt and Arthur L. Caplan, eds, *Scientific Controversies: Case Studies in the Resolution and Closure of Disputes in Science and Technology* (Cambridge: Cambridge University Press, 1987), especially Ronald Bayer, 'Politics, Science and the Problem of Psychiatric Nomenclature: A Case Study of the American Psychiatric Association Referendum on Homosexuality,' 381–400; Robert L. Spitzer, 'The Diagnostic Studies of Homosexuality in DSM-III: A Reformulation of the Issues,' 401–16; and Irving

Bieber, 'On Arriving at the American Psychiatric Association Decision on Homosexuality,' 417–36.

50 See, for example, Fiona A. K. Campbell, 'Inciting Legal Fictions: "Disability's" Date with Ontology and the Ableist Body of the Law,' *Griffith Law Review* 10 (2001): 42–62.

51 See, for example, B.P. Tucker, 'Deaf Culture, Cochlear Implants, and Elective Disability,' *Hastings Center Report* 28 (1998): 6–14.

52 See, for example, Mariamne H. Whatley, 'The Picture of Health: How Textbook Photographs Construct Health,' in *The Ideology of Images in Educational Media: Hidden Curriculums in the Classroom*, ed. Elizabeth Ellsworth and Mariamne H. Whatley (New York and London: Teachers College of Columbia University, 1990), 121–40.

53 Ann Lukits, 'The Growing Numbers of Flat-Headed Babies,' *Kingston Whig-Standard*, 10 August 2002, 1, 11.

Chapter 2: Lovers: The Rise and Apparent Fall of Lovesickness

1 Dean H. Hamer, 'Sexual Orientation [letter].' *Nature Neuroscience* 365 (1993): 702; Dean H. Hamer, S. Hu, V.L. Magnuson, N. Hu, and A.M. Pattatucci, 'A Linkage between DNA Markers on the X Chromosome and Male Sexual Orientation,' *Science* 261 (1993): 321–7.

2 Ingrid Wickelgren, 'Discovery of "Gay Gene" Questioned,' *Science* 284 (1999): 571; G. Rice, C. Anderson, N. Risch, and G. Ebers, 'Male Homosexuality: Absence of Linkage to Microsatellite Markers at Xq28,' *Science* 284 (1999): 665–7; Jocelyn Kaiser, 'No Misconduct in "Gay Gene" Study,' *Science* 275 (1997): 1251; Eliot Marshall, 'NIH's "Gay Gene" Study Questioned,' *Science* 268 (1995): 1841.

3 On this discovery and the public reaction to it, see Chandler Burr, *A Separate Creation: The Search for the Biological Origins of Sexual Orientation* (New York: Hyperion, 1996), esp. 198–205.

4 Ted Peters, 'On the "Gay Gene": Back to Original Sin Again?' *Dialog: A Journal of Theology* 33 (1994): 30–8.

5 Udo Schüklenk, Edward Stein, Jacinta Kerin, and William Byne, 'The Ethics of Genetic Research on Sexual Orientation,' *Hastings Center Report* 27 (1997): 6–13.

6 Diane Ackerman, *A Natural History of Love* (New York: Vintage Books, 1994), xix; Rosemary Sullivan, *Labyrinth of Desire: A Story of*

Women and Romantic Obsession (Toronto: Harper Collins Flamingo
Canada, 2001), 2.

7 Linda Phyllis Austern, 'Musical Treatments for Lovesickness,' in
Music as Medicine: The History of Music Therapy since Antiquity, ed.
Peregrine Horden (Aldershot: Ashgate, 2000), 213–45; Bill Bynum,
'Discarded Diagnoses: Lovesickness,' *Lancet* 357 (2001): 403; Adel-
heid Giedke, 'Die Liebeskrankheit in der Geschichte der Medizin,'
dissertation zur Erlangung des Grades eines Doktors der Medizin,
Universität Düsseldorf aus dem Institut für Geschichte der
Medizin, 1983; John Livingston Lowes, 'The Loveres Maladye of
Hereos,' *Modern Philology* 11 (1913–14): 491–546; Michael R.
McVaugh, 'Introduction,' in *Arnaldi De Villanova Opera Medica
Omnia,* vol. 3, ed. Michael R. McVaugh (Barcelona: Universitat de
Barcelona, 1985), 11–39; Einar Petterson, *Amans Amanti Medicus: Das
Genremotiv der ärtztliche Besuch in seinem kulturhistorischen Kontext*
(Berlin: Gabr. Mann Verlag, 2000), 282–314; J.M. Schneck, 'The Love-
Sick Patient in the History of Medicine,' *Journal of the History of
Medicine and Allied Sciences* 12 (1957): 266–7; Reay Tannahill, *Sex
in History* (New York: Stein and Day, 1980); Mary Frances Wack,
Lovesickness in the Middle Ages: The Viaticum and Its Commentaries
(Philadelphia: University of Pennsylvania Press, 1990), 3–30.

8 Bernadette Brooten, *Love between Women: Early Christian Responses to
Female Homoeroticism* (Chicago and London: University of Chicago
Press, 1996).

9 Vernon A. Rosario, *The Erotic Imagination: French Histories of Perver-
sity* (New York and Oxford: Oxford University Press, 1997); A.L.
Rowse, *Homosexuals in History: A Study of Ambivalence in Society,
Literature, and the Arts* (New York: Macmillan, 1977).

10 Peter Lewis Allen, *The Wages of Sin: Sex and Disease, Past and Present*
(Chicago: University of Chicago Press, 2000).

11 Stanley W. Jackson, *Melancholia and Depression: From Hippocratic
Times to Modern Times* (New Haven: Yale University Press, 1986),
352–73; Raymond Klibansky, Erwin Panofsky, and Fritz Saxl, *Saturn
and Melancholy: Studies in the History of Natural Philosophy, Religion,
and Art* (Cambridge and London: Nelson, 1964); Jean Starobinski,
Histoire de la traitement de la mélancholie des origines à 1900 (Basel: J.R.
Geigy, *Acta Psychosomatica,* 4, 1960).

12 I am not the first to have made this observation. It is dealt with in great detail by Darryl W. Amundsen, 'Romanticizing the Ancient Medical Profession,' *Bulletin of the History of Medicine* 48 (1974): 328–37; Hans-Hinrich Biesterfeldt and Dimitri Gutas, 'The Malady of Love,' *Journal of the American Oriental Society* 104 (1984): 21–55; Massimo Ciavolella, *La malattia d'amore dall'antichità al medioevo* (Rome: Bulzoni, 1976); Marie-Paule Duminil, 'La mélancholie amoureuse dans l'antiquité,' in *La folie et le corps*, ed. J. Céard (Paris: Presses de l'École Normale Supérieure, 1985), 91–110; Hermann Funke, 'Greische und römische Antike,' in *Liebe als Krankheit. 3 Kolloquium der Forschungsstelle für Europäishe lyrik des Mittelalters*, ed. Theo Stemmler (Mannheim and Tübingen: Narr and Universität Mannheim, 1990), 11–30; Adelheid Giedke, 'Die Liebeskrankheit in der Geschichte der Medizin,' 1983; Bernhard D. Haage, '"Amor hereos" als medizinischer terminus technicus in der Antike und im Mittelalter,' in *Liebe als Krankheit*, ed. Stemmler, 31–74; Klibansky et al., *Saturn and Melancholy*; Richard Walzer, 'Aristotle, Galen, and Palladius on Love,' in *Greek into Arabic: Essays on Islamic Philosophy*, Oriental Studies, vol. 1, ed. S.M. Stern and Richard Walzer (Oxford: Bruno Cassirer, [1939] 1963), 48–60.

13 R.O. Faulkner, Edward F. Wente, and William Kelly Simpson, eds, *The Literature of Ancient Egypt* (New Haven and London: Yale University Press, 1973), 298, 300; Ezra Pound and Noel Stock, *Love Poems of Ancient Egypt* (New York: New Directions, 1976 [1962]). See also an Egyptian poem cited in Amundsen, 'Romanticizing,' 332.

14 Hesiod, 'Theogony,' in *Hesiod*, trans. Richmond Lattimore (Ann Arbor: University of Michigan Press, 1959), 119–86, esp. 130, lines 120–2.

15 Sappho, 'Lovesickness, an Echo of Sappho by Theocritus [Wharton 167; Edmonds 189],' in *Songs of Sappho, Including the Recent Egyptian Discoveries*, ed. and trans. Marion Mills Miller and David M. Robinson (Lexington, KY: Maxwelton Company, 1925), 98; See also Sappho, *If Not, Winter: Fragments of Sappho*, ed. and trans. Anne Carson (New York: Alfred A. Knopf, 2002), 121 ('all my skin old age already') and 265 ('Eros the melter of limbs').

16 Sappho, *If Not, Winter*, trans. Carson, 63; see also 77 ('you burn me').

For another translation of the same fragment, see Amundsen, 'Romanticizing,' 331–2.

17 For more on lovesickness in ancient Greek poetry, see Anne Carson, *Eros the Bittersweet* (Princeton: Princeton University Press, 1986) and Monica Silveira Cyrino, *In Pandora's Jar: Lovesickness in Early Greek Poetry* (Lanham, MD: University Press of America, 1995).

18 See Homer, *Odyssey*, Book 5 (Odysseus weeping for home) and Book 20 (Penelope weeping for her husband and imploring the gods to end her life). *The Odyssey of Homer*, trans. and ed. Richmond Lattimore (New York: Harper Row, 1965, 1967), 90, 299–30.

19 Hermann Funke, 'Greische und römische Antike'; Benedikt Konrad Vollmann, 'Liebe als Krankheit in der weltlichen Lyrik des lateinischen Mittelalters,' in *Liebe als Krankheit*, ed. Stemmler, 105–25; Marilyn B. Skinner, 'Disease Imagery in Catullus,' *Classical Philology* 82 (1987): 230–3.

20 Ovid, 'Remedia amoris,' in *Ovid in Six Volumes*, trans. J.H. Mozley (Cambridge, MA, and London: Harvard University Press and Heinemann, 1979), 2: 178–233. See also Lenz, *Ovid. Heilmittel gegen die Liebe*.

21 Ovid, 'Remedia amoris' (lines 717–19), 226–7.

22 Ibid. (line 535), 214–15.

23 Ibid. (lines 403–5), 204–5.

24 Ibid. (line 317), 198–201.

25 Ibid. (lines 411–39), 206–7.

26 Ibid. (line 525), 212–13.

27 Ibid. (lines 92–3), 184–5.

28 Ibid. (line 313), 198–9.

29 Marcus Tullius Cicero, 'Tusculan Disputationes IV,' in *Tusculan Disputationes*, Loeb Classical Library, trans. J.E. King (Cambridge, MA, and London: Harvard University Press and Heinemann, 1971), 8: 326–423, especially sections 26–31 (on sickness and disease), 352–9; sections 65–76 (on love), 402–15; section 74 (on its treatment), 412–13. The quotation is on 411. On Aristotle's views and his vanished treatise 'Erotikos,' see Walzer, 'Aristotle, Galen, and Palladius on Love.'

30 Theophrastus, cited in Walzer, 'Aristotle, Galen, and Palladius on Love,' 58.

31 Erasistratus, the famous Alexandrian physician of the third century
BC, is identified in the versions of Galen and Plutarch. In Lucian's
version the young man's disease stems from guilt as well as love.
Galen, *Galeni de Praecognitionae. Galen on Prognosis. Edition, Transla-
tion, and Commentary*, ed. Vivian Nutton (Berlin: Corpus Medicorum
Grecorum V 8, 1; Akademie Verlag, 1979), 100–1; Plutarch, 'Demetrius,' in *Plutarch's Lives*, trans. J. Langhorne and W. Langhorne
(London: J.J. Chidley, 1842), 941–66, esp. 958–9; Lucian, *The Syrian
Goddess (De dea Syria)* (Missoula, MT: Scholars Press for the Society
of Biblical Literature, 1976), passages 17, 18, on 24–9. A similar
doctor's ploy was told by the fifth-century AD writer of fiction,
Aristainetos. For a translation, see Amundsen, 'Romanticizing,'
329–31.

32 J.E.D. Esquirol, *Mental Maladies. A Treatise on Insanity*, trans. E.K.
Hunt (New York and London: Hafner, [1845] 1965), 339. See also
Gaspard Caldera de Heredia, *Tribunal medicum, magicum, et politicum. De prognosi fallacia in communi et particulari* (Lugduni Batavorum: Joannes Elsevierum, 1658); André Du Laurens, *Les oeuvres
de M. André Dulaurens*, 2 parts in one volume (Paris: Nicolas et
Jean Lacoste, 1646), pt. 2, chap. 3, 'maladies mélancholiques,' 309;
J.D. Gaub's essay of 1763, in L.J. Rather, *Mind and Body in Eighteenth-Century Medicine: A Study Based on Jerome Gaub's 'De regimine
mentis'* (London: The Wellcome Historical Medical Library, 1965),
150.

33 Carol Merriam, 'Clinical Cures for Love in Propertius' *Elegies,' Scholia: Studies in Classical Antiquity* 10 (2001): 69–76.

34 Sextus Propertius, *The Poems of Sextus Propertius*, trans. J.P. McCulloch (Berkeley: University of California Press, 1972), book II, poem
1, 59–60.

35 Hippocrates, 'Affections' and 'Regimen in Acute Diseases,' in
Hippocrates with an English Translation. Loeb Classical Library, 8 vols,
trans. Paul Potter (Cambridge, MA: Harvard University Press 1988),
5: 7, and 6: 303–5, respectively. On young girls, see Hippocrate, 'Des
maladies des jeunes filles,' in *Oeuvres complètes d'Hippocrate*, vol. 8,
trans. E. Littré (Paris: Baillière, 1853); Mary R. Lefkowitz and Maureen B. Fant, *Women's Life in Greece and Rome: A Source Book in Translation* (London: Duckworth, 1992), 242–3. See also E.D. Baumann,

'Die pseudohippokratische Schrift "Peri Manies,"' *Janus* 42 (1938): 129–41.

36 Thought by other doctors to have been consumptive, the young man's tell-tale blushing at the sight of his father's concubine Phila led Hippocrates to 'diagnose' lovesickness instead of disease. Jody Rubin Pinault, *Hippocratic Lives and Legends* (London: E.J. Brill, 1992), 61–77.

37 Galen, *De propriorum animi cujusque affectuum dignotione et curatione. On the Passions and Errors of the Soul* (Columbus: Ohio State University Press, 1963), 32.

38 Galen, *De locis affectis. On the Affected Parts* (Basel: Karger, 1976), book 6, chap. 5, 184.

39 Galen, *Galeni de praecognitionae*, chap. 6, 100–6. See also Galen, 'Galeni de praenotione ad Posthumum liber,' *Opera Omnia*, ed. C.G. Kuhn (Hildesheim: Georg Olms, 1965), 14: 630–5. See also Amundsen, 'Romanticizing,' 335–6; and Arthur John Brock, *Greek Medicine, Being Extracts Illustrative of Medical Writers from Hippocrates to Galen* (London: J.M. Dent and Sons, 1929), 213–14.

40 Aretaeus, 'Chronic Diseases, Book I,' in *Extant Works of Aretaeus the Cappadocian*, trans. F. Adams (London: Sydenham Society, 1856), 298–300.

41 As for the cure of melancholy, Aretaeus recommended bleeding, cupping, wormwood, diet, frictions, and baths, but he did not refer to love, sex, or other behaviours. Ibid.

42 W.W. Fortenbaugh, *Aristotle on Emotions* (London: Duckworth, 1975); Walzer, 'Aristotle, Galen, and Palladius on Love.' For a general introduction to Aristotle on the soul, see Philip J. Van der Eijk, 'Aristotle's Psycho-Physiological Account of the Soul-Body Relationship,' in *Psyche and Soma: Physicians and Metaphysicians on the Mind-Body Problem from Antiquity to Enlightenment*, ed. John Wright and Paul Potter (Oxford: Clarendon Oxford University Press, 2000), 57–77.

43 For a fascinating account of why disorders of affect are less attended to than disorders of cognition or intellect, see G.E. Berrios, 'The Psychopathology of Affectivity: Conceptual and Historical Aspects,' *Psychological Medicine* 15 (1985): 745–58.

44 Oribase, 'Des amoureux,' in *Oeuvres d'Oribase en 6 volumes*, trans.

U.C. Bussemaker and C. Daremberg (Paris: Baillière, 1851–76), vol. 5 (1873), 413–4. For more on Oribasius, see Mark Grant, *Dieting for an Emperor. A Translation of Books 1 and 4 of Oribasius' Medical Compilations with an Introduction and Commentary*, Studies in Ancient Medicine, Vol. 15, ed. John Scarborough (Leiden: Brill, 1997).

45 Oribase, 'Des amoureux,' 414.

46 On the history of pulse as a diagnostic sign for love, see Marek-Marsel Mesulam and Jon Perry, 'The Diagnosis of Love-Sickness: Experimental Psychophysiology with the Polygraph,' *Psychophysiology* 9 (1972): 546–51.

47 Paulus Aegineta, 'On Lovesick Persons,' in *The Seven Books of Paulus Aegineta*, trans. F. Adams (London: New Sydenham Society, 1844–7), 1: 390–1.

48 Caelius Aurelianus, *De morbis acutis; De morbis chronicas. On Acute Diseases and On Chronic Diseases*, trans. I.E. Drabkin (Chicago: University of Chicago Press, 1950), 556–9.

49 Saint Paul was not the first to make these distinctions. Contemporary Roman religion recognized several gods in the domain of love, such as Venus, Cupid, and Priapus, to name only three. Granted, they were deities not demons. Nevertheless, Paul has been heavily criticized for subsequent interpretations of his words. See, for example, Allen, *The Wages of Sin*, 17.

50 Rhazes, 'De coturub vel eros,' in *Continens, liber primus*, Tractatus 20, cited in Biesterfeldt and Gutas, 'The Malady of Love.'

51 Avicenna (Ibn Sina), 'De Ilisci. Insania ex amoribus,' *Liber Canonis de Medicinis*, Liber 3, Tract 4, cap 22 (Brussels: Éditions Culture et Civilisation, facsimile of Venice 1527 edition ed., 1971), 151v–152r.

52 Walzer, 'Aristotle, Galen, and Palladius on Love.'

53 Mary Frances Wack, 'The *Liber de heros morbo* of Johannes Afflacius and Its Implications for Medieval Love Conventions,' *Speculum* 62 (1987): 324–44

54 Danielle Jacquart and Claude Thomasset, *Sexuality and Medicine in the Middle Ages*, trans. Matthew Adamson (Princeton: Princeton University Press, 1988), 130; Wack, *Lovesickness in the Middle Ages*, 41. On the rules governing Christian Europe, see the learned essays by James A. Brundage, *Sex, Law, and Marriage in the Middle Ages* (Aldershot, UK, and Brookfield, VT: Ashgate, 1993).

55 Biesterfeldt and Gutas, 'The Malady of Love'; J.C. Bürgel, 'Love, Lust, and Longing: Eroticism in Early Islam as Reflected in Literary Sources,' in *Sixth Giorgio Levi della Vida Biennial Conference Society and the Sexes in Medieval Islam*, ed. A.L. al-Sayyid-Marsot (Malibu: Undena Press, 1979), 81–117; Johann Christoph Bürgel, 'Der Topos der Liebeskrankheit in der klassichen Dichtung des Islam,' in *Liebe als Krankheit*, ed. Stemmler, 75–104; A.E. Khairallah, *Love, Madness, and Poetry: An Interpretation of the Magnun Legend* (Beirut: Beiruter Texte und Studien, Band 25, 1980).

56 Stith Thompson, *Motif-Index of Folk-Literature*, 6 vols (Bloomington: Indiana University Press, 1955–8), 5: 335–6, 346–7.

57 Wack, *Lovesickness in the Middle Ages*.

58 Constantine the African, 'Viaticum I.20 [ca. 1180–1200],' in Wack, *Lovesickness in the Middle Ages*, 179–93.

59 On medieval attitudes to sexuality among clerics and peasants, see Jacquart and Thomasset, *Sexuality and Medicine in the Middle Ages*; Emannuel Le Roy Ladurie, *Montaillou, village occitan de 1294 à 1324* (Paris: Gallimard, 1975).

60 On Rufus, see Michael R. McVaugh, 'Introduction,' in *Arnaldi de Villanova Opera Medica Omnia*, 3: 16–17; Biesterfeldt and Gutas, 'The Malady of Love.'

61 Danielle Jacquart, 'L'amour "héroique" à travers le traité d'Arnaud de Villeneuve,' in *La folie et le corps*, ed. Céard, 143–58; Jacquart and Thomasset, *Sexuality and Medicine in the Middle Ages*, 133–4; Lowes, 'The Loveres Maladye of Hereos,' 491–546; Michael R. McVaugh, *Medicine before the Plague: Practitioners and Their Patients in the Crown of Aragon, 1285–1345* (Cambridge: Cambridge University Press, 1993), 201; John M. Steadman, 'Courtly Love as a Problem of Style,' in *Chaucer und seine Zeit. Symposium für Walter F. Schirmer*, ed. Arno Esch (Tübingen: Max Niemyer Verlag, 1968), 1–33, esp. 23–4; Wack, 'The *Liber de Heros Morbo* of Johannes Afflacius'; Wack, *Lovesickness in the Middle Ages*, 182–5.

62 Arnaldus de Villanova, 'Tractatus de amore heroico [ca 1280],' in *Arnaldi de Villanova Opera Medica Omnia*, ed. R. McVaugh, 3: 1–54; McVaugh, *Medicine before the Plague*, 201.

63 Nancy G. Siraisi, *Medieval and Early Renaissance Medicine: An Introduction to Knowledge and Practice* (Chicago: University of Chicago Press, 1990), 131.

64 Rüdiger Schnell, *Causa amoris. Liebeskonzeption und Liebesdarstellung in der mittelalterlichen Literatur* (Bern and Munich: Francke Verlag, 1985); Werner Hoffman, 'Liebe als Krankheit in der mittelhochdeutschen Lyrik,' in *Liebe als Krankheit*, ed. Stemmler, 221–57; Friedrich Wolfzettel, 'Liebe als Krankheit in der altfranzösischen Literatur,' in *Liebe als Krankheit*, ed. Stemmler, 151–86; Karl Reichl, 'Liebe als Krankheit: mittelenglische Texte,' in *Liebe als Krankheit*, ed. Stemmler, 187–220; Rupprecht Rohr, 'Liebe als Krankheit bei den Troubadors,' in *Liebe als Krankheit*, ed. Stemmler, 139–50; Michael Solomon, *The Literature of Misogyny in Medieval Spain: The 'Archipreste de Talavera' and the 'Spill'* (New York and Cambridge: Cambridge University Press, 1997), esp. 17–64.

65 Julia Blanco Fernández, 'El amor hereos en La Celestina: la prescripción de Celestina' (MA thesis, McGill University, 1999); Michael Calabrese, 'The Lover's Cure in Ovid's *Remedia amoris* and Chaucer's *Miller's Tale*,' *English Language Notes* 32 (1994): 13–18; Peter Dronke, *Medieval Latin and the Rise of the European Love-Lyric* (Oxford: Clarendon, 1968); Marie-Madeleine Fontaine, 'La lignée des commentaires à la chanson de Guido Cavalcanti "Donna me prega": évolution des relations entre philosophie, médecine, et littérature dans le débat sur la nature d'amour (de la fin de XIIIe siècle à celle du XVIe),' in *La folie et le corps*, ed. Céard, 159–78; Carol Falvo Hefferman, *The Melancholy Muse: Chaucer, Shakespeare, and Early Medicine* (Pittsburgh: Duquesnne University Press, 1995); Robert Hollander, *Boccaccio's Two Venuses* (New York: Columbia University Press, 1977); Lloyd Howard, 'Dino's Interpretation of "Donna me prega" and Cavalcanti's "Canzoniere,"' *Canadian Journal of Italian Studies* 6 (1983): 167–82; C.S. Lewis, *The Allegory of Love: A Study in Medieval Tradition* (Oxford and New York: Oxford University Press, 1936, 1990); Steadman, 'Courtly Love as a Problem of Style'; Mary Frances Wack, 'Memory and Love in Chaucer's "Troilus and Criseyde"' (thesis, Cornell University, 1982); Mary Frances Wack, 'From Mental Faculties to Magical Philters: The Entry of Magic into Academic Medical Writing on Lovesickness, 13th–17th Centuries,' in *Eros and Anteros: The Medical Traditions of Love in the Renaissance*, ed. Donald Beecher and Massimo Ciavolella, University of Toronto Italian Studies no. 9 (Ottawa: Dovehouse Press, 1992), 9–31.

66 For example, see Howard, 'Dino's Interpretation'; Massimo Cia-

volella, 'Mediaeval Medicine and Arcite's Love Sickness,' *Florilegium* 1 (1979): 222–41.

67 Joan Tasker Grimbert, '*Voleir* vs. *Poeir*: Frustrated Desire in Thomas's *Tristan*,' *Philological Quarterly* 69 (1990): 153–65; Alfred Karnein, 'Amor est passio: A Definition of Courtly Love,' in *Court and Poet: Selected Proceedings of the Third Congress of the International Courtly Literature Society*, ed. Glynn S. Burgess (Liverpool: Francis Cairns, 1981), 215–21; Lewis, *Allegory of Love*; Schnell, *Causa amoris*; Steadman, 'Courtly Love as a Problem of Style.'

68 Andreas Capellanus, *De amore. Andreas Capellanus on Love*, ed. G. Walsh (Worcester and London: Trinity Press, 1982); Karnein, 'Amor est passio'; Lewis, *Allegory of Love*; Steadman, 'Courtly Love as a Problem of Style.'

69 Capellanus, *De amore*, 147–57.

70 Ibid., 286–305.

71 Ibid., 306–25.

72 Jacquart and Thomasset, *Sexuality and Medicine*, 96–100.

73 For a concise introduction to early modern nosology, see Lester S. King, *Medical Thinking: A Historical Preface* (Princeton: Princeton University Press, 1982), 117–23.

74 Girolamo Fracastoro, *Syphilis, or the French Disease*, trans. Heneage Wynne-Finch (London: Heinemann, 1935), 101–3.

75 Jacques Ferrand, *A Treatise on Lovesickness*, ed. and trans. Donald A. Beecher and Massimo Ciavolella (Syracuse: Syracuse University Press, 1990).

76 Donald Beecher, 'Erotic Love and the Inquisition: Jacques Ferrand and the Tribunal of Toulouse, 1620,' *The Sixteenth Century Journal* 20 (1989): 41–53.

77 Daniel Sennert, 'Institutionum medicinae,' in *Opera* (Lugduni: Joannes Autorii Huguetan, 1656), vol. 2, tome 3, 'De capitis cum internorum tum externorum motus que spontanei u. affectionibus,' pt II, 'De symptomatibus quae in sensibus internis et cerebro accidunt,' cap. X, 'Amore insano,' 94–7.

78 André Du Laurens, *Les oeuvres de M. André Du Laurens*, part 2, chap. 3, 'Discours sur la conservation de la vue, des maladies mélancholiques, etc,' sections X and XI, 308–11.

79 Francesco Guardiani, 'Eros and Misogyny from Giovan Battista

Marino to Ferrante Pallavicino,' in *Eros and Anteros*, ed. Beecher and Ciavolella, 147–59.

80 David Gentilcore, 'Ritualized Illness and Music Therapy: Views of Tarantism in the Kingdom of Naples,' in *Music as Medicine*, ed. Horden, 256–72. On narcissism, see the 1646 case history of 'a gentleman,' Du Laurens, *Oeuvres*, 309.

81 Karl Figlio, 'Chlorosis and Chronic Disease in Nineteenth-Century Britain: The Social Construction of Somatic Illness in a Capitalist Society,' *Social History* 3 (1978): 167–97; Robert Hudson, 'The Biography of Disease: Lessons from Chlorosis,' *Bulletin of the History of Medicine* 51 (1977): 448–63; Helen King, '"Green Sickness": Hippocrates, Galen, and the Origins of the Disease of Virgins,' *International Journal of the Classical Tradition* 2 (1996): 372–87; Irvine Loudon, 'The Disease Called Chlorosis,' *Psychological Medicine* 14 (1984): 27–36; Irvine S. Loudon, 'Chlorosis, Anaemia, and Anorexia Nervosa,' *British Medical Journal* 281 (1980): 1669–75.

82 Jackie Pigeaud, 'Reflections on Love-Melancholy in Robert Burton,' trans. Faith Wallis, in *Eros and Anteros*, ed. Beecher and Ciavolella (1992), 211–31.

83 More than eighty such images are reproduced in Petterson, *Amans Amanti Medicus*.

84 Linda Phyllis Austern, '"For Love's a Good Musician": Performance, Audition, and Erotic Disorders in Early Modern Europe,' *Musical Quarterly* 82 (1998): 614–53.

85 Roy Porter, 'The Literature of Sexual Advice before 1800,' *Sexual Knowledge, Sexual Science: The History of Attitudes to Sexuality*, ed. Roy Porter and Mikuláš Teich (Cambridge: Cambridge University Press, 1994), 134–57.

86 Voltaire, *Dictionnaire philosophique* (Paris: Garnier-Flammarion, [1764] 1964), 34–5; M. Levor, 'Die Liebeskrankheit in Goethes Dichtung,' *Deutsche Medizinische Wochenschrift* 37 (1911): 220–2; Mary-Beth Gugler, 'Mercury and the "Pains of Love" in Jonathan Swift's "A Beautiful Young Nymph Going to Bed,"' *English Language Notes* 20 (1991): 31–6.

87 The short thesis was reprinted in Latin in 1963. François Boissier de Sauvages, 'Dissertatio medica atque ludicra de amore. Utrum sit amor medicabilis herbis? [1724]' *Monspeliensis Hippocrates* 20 (été

1963): 10–15. This reprint was based on an early nineteenth-century edition of what was almost certainly a manuscript thesis. Neither the original manuscript, nor the early nineteenth-century edition can now be traced. I am grateful to Mireille Vial and her colleagues at the Bibliothèque de l'École de Médecine de Montpellier for attempting to locate these works.

88 François Boissier de Sauvages, *Pathologia methodica, seu de cognoscendis morbis* (Amstelodami: Sumptibus Fratrum de Tournes, 1752), 241–3; François Boissier de Sauvages, *Pathologia methodica, seu de cognoscendis morbis,* tertia ed. (Lugduni: Typis Petri de Bruyset: Fratrum de Tournes, 1759), 345–50; François Boissier de Sauvages, *Nosologia methodica,* 2 vols (Amstelodami: Sumptibus Fratrum de Tournes, 1768), vol. 2, 252–3 (erotomania). For more on Sauvages, see Lester S. King, 'Boissier de Sauvages and 18th-Century Nosology,' *Bulletin of the History of Medicine* 40 (1966): 43–51; Julian Martin, 'Sauvages's Nosology: Medical Enlightenment in Montpellier,' *The Medical Enlightenment of the Eighteenth Century,* ed. Andrew Cunningham and Roger K. French (Cambridge: Cambridge University Press, 1990), 111–37.

89 Hieronymus David Gaubius, 'Pathologia specialis,' article #542, in *Institutiones pathologiae medicinalis* (Lipsiae: Joannis Pauli Krausii Bibliopolae Viennensis, 1759), 278. For a translation and commentary on another essay by Gaub on lovesickness, see Rather, *Mind and Body,* 149–52.

90 William Cullen, *Apparatus ad nosologiam methodicam seu Synopsis nosologiae methodicae in usu studiosorum* (Amstelodami: Fratrum de Tournes, 1775), 58 (for erotomania according to Linnaeus) and 220 (Cullen). Another nosologist, J.B. Sagar, did not include a category for erotomania, although he classified separate disease entities for nymphomania, satyriasis, priapism, and anaphrodisia. Johann Baptist Michael Sagar, *Systema morborum symptomaticum secundum classes, ordines, genera et species,* 2 vols (Vienna: J.P. Krause, 1771). For more on lovesickness in the early modern period, see Adelheid Giedke, 'Die Liebeskrankheit in der Geschichte der Medizin.'

91 *Merchant of Venice* 3.2.63–4.

92 Esquirol, *Mental Maladies,* 335–42. Esquirol also recognized a form

of melancholy that was 'not a disease' (335), which he described in detail in a chapter on 'lypemania' or melancholy (229–31).

93 Jean-Nicolas Corvisart des Marets, *An Essay on the Organic Diseases and Lesions of the Heart and Great Vessels*, trans. Jacob Gates (New York: Hafner Publishing House, [1806] 1962), 275.

94 Henri Marie Beyle [Stendhal], *De l'amour/Love*, trans. Gilbert Sale, Suzanne Sale, and Jean Stewart (London: Penguin, [1822] 1975).

95 On the history of masturbation as a disease, see H.T. Englehardt, 'The Disease of Masturbation: Values and the Concept of Disease,' *Bulletin of the History of Medicine* 48 (1974): 234–48; Fernando Vidal, 'An 18th-Century Debate about Masturbation and Lust in Young Children,' unpublished paper, read at 'Health and the Child: Care and Culture in History,' Geneva, 13–15 September 2001.

96 Rosario, *The Erotic Imagination*; Allen, *Wages of Sin*.

97 Helen Small, *Love's Madness: Medicine, the Novel, and Female Insanity, 1800–1865* (Oxford: Clarendon Press, 1996); Athena Vrettos, *Somatic Fictions: Imagining Illness in Victorian Culture* (Stanford, CA: Stanford University Press, 1995).

98 Bram Dijkstra, *Idols of Perversity: Fantasies of Feminine Evil in Fin-de-Siècle Culture* (New York and Oxford: Oxford University Press, 1986), esp. 25–35.

99 Bert Hansen, 'American Physicians' "Discovery" of Homosexuals, 1880–1900: A New Diagnosis in a Changing Society,' in *Framing Disease: Studies in Cultural History*, ed. Charles E. Rosenberg and Janet Golden (New Brunswick, NJ: Rutgers University Press, 1992), 104–33.

100 Judith Walzer Leavitt, *Brought to Bed: Childbearing in America, 1750 to 1950* (New York: Oxford University Press, 1986).

101 Wendy Mitchinson, *The Nature of Their Bodies: Women and Their Doctors in Victorian Canada* (Toronto: University of Toronto Press, 1991), 252–77.

102 Berrios, 'Psychopathology of Affectivity.'

103 J. Miriam Benn, *The Predicaments of Love* (London: Pluto Press, 1992); Alexander C.T. Geppert, 'Divine Sex, Happy Marriage, Regenerated Nation: Marie Stopes's Marital Manual *Married Love* and the Making of a Best-Seller,' *Journal of the History of Sexuality* 8 (1998): 389–433; Ivan Crozier, '"Rough Winds Do Shake the Dar-

ling Buds of May": William Acton and the Sexuality of the Child,'
unpublished paper read at 'Health and the Child: Care and Culture in History,' Geneva, 13–15 September 2001. On Wells, see A.B.
McKillop, *The Spinster and the Prophet: Florence Deeks, H.G. Wells,
and the Mystery of the Purloined Past* (Toronto: Macfarlane Walter
and Ross, 2001), esp. 169–70 (on his relationship with Sanger).

104 Alfred C. Kinsey, *Sexual Behavior in the Human Male* (Philadephia:
Saunders, 1948); Alfred C. Kinsey, *Sexual Behavior in the Human
Female* (Philadelphia: Saunders, 1953); William H. Masters and Virginia E. Johnson, *Human Sexual Response* (Boston: Little, Brown,
1966); Shere Hite, *The Hite Report: A Nationwide Study on Female
Sexuality* (New York: Macmillan, 1976); Shere Hite, *The Hite Report
on Male Sexuality* (New York: Knopf, 1981).

105 Pierre Léger, *La canadienne française et l'amour, ou l'homme démystifié*
(Montreal: Éditions du jour, 1965).

106 Alex Comfort, ed., *The Joy of Sex: A Cordon Bleu Guide to Lovemaking*
(New York: Simon and Schuster, 1972); Alex Comfort, ed., *The Joy
of Sex: A Gourmet Guide to Lovemaking* (New York: Crown Publishers, 1972).

107 Dr Jocelyn Elders spoke in the context of alternative sexual practices for avoiding AIDS. In the ensuing furor, President Bill Clinton
asked for and received her resignation. She had been the first black
women to serve as Surgeon General. Daniel Greenberg, 'Out Goes
the Surgeon General,' *Lancet* 344 (1994): 1760.

108 E-mail sent to a Queen's University list-serve by a staff member,
'Hello from the Ban Righ Centre,' 16 August 2002.

109 Dr John Bradford, 'Pedophilia: Horrifying: But Is It a Crime?' *Globe
and Mail*, 20 November 2000, A19.

110 Jonas E. Salk, 'Biological Basis of Disease and Behaviour,' *Perspectives in Biology and Medicine* 5 (1962): 198–206. See also G.F. Solomon and R.F. Moos, 'Emotions, Immunity, and Disease,' *Archives
of General Psychiatry* 11 (1964): 657. Similar studies have addressed
the social function of pain, for example, Wulf Schiefenhovel, 'Perception, Expression, and Social Function of Pain: A Human Ethological View,' *Science in Context* 8 (1995): 31–46.

111 Candace B. Pert and Solomon H. Snyder, 'Opiate Receptor: Demonstration in Nervous Tissue,' *Science* 179 (1973): 1011–14. On this

discovery and its implications, see Jeff Goldberg, *Anatomy of a Scientific Discovery* (Toronto and New York: Bantam, 1988).

112 Douglas A. Drossman, Jane Leserman, Ginette Nachman, Zhiming Li, Honi Gluck, Timothy C. Tommey, and C. Madeline Mitchell, 'Sexual and Physical Abuse in Women with Functional or Organic Gastrointestinal Disorders,' *Annals of Internal Medicine* 113 (1990): 828–33; Douglas A. Drossman, Nicholas J. Talley, Jane Leserman, Kevin W. Olden, and Marcelo A. Barreiro, 'Sexual and Physical Abuse in Gastrointestinal Illness: Review and Recommendations,' *Annals of Internal Medicine* 123 (1995): 782–94; Joanna M. Hill, William L. Farrar, and Candace B. Pert, 'Autoradiographic Localization of T4 Antigen, the HIV Receptor, in Human Brain,' *International Journal of Neuroscience* 32 (1987): 687–93.

113 Mark L. Laudenslager, Susan M. Ryan, Richard Hyson, and Steven F. Maier, 'Coping and Immunosuppression: Inescapable but Not Escapable Shock Suppresses Lymphocyte Proliferation,' *Science* 221 (1983): 568–70; M.E. Lewis, M. Mishkin, E. Bragin, R.M. Brown, C.B. Pert, and A. Pert, 'Opiate Receptor Gradients in Monkey Cerebral Cortex: Correspondence with Sensory Processing Hierarchies,' *Science* 211 (1981): 1166–9; Yehuda Shavit, James W. Lewis, Robert Gale, and John C. Lieberskind, 'Opioid Peptides Mediate the Suppressive Effect of Stress on Natural Killer Cell Cytotoxicity,' *Science* 223 (1984): 188–90; L.S. Sklar and H. Anisman, 'Stress and Coping Factors Influence Tumor Growth,' *Science* 205 (1979): 513–15.

114 Candace B. Pert, Michael R. Ruff, Richard J. Weber, and Miles Herkenham, 'Neuropeptides and Their Receptors,' *Journal of Immunology* 135, no. 2, Supplement (1985), 820s–6s; Candace B. Pert, *Molecules of Emotion: Why You Feel the Way You Feel* (New York: Scribner, 1997); Candace B. Pert, Henry E. Dreher, and Michael R. Ruff, 'The Psychosomatic Network: Foundations of Mind-Body Medicine,' *Alternative Therapies in Health and Medicine* 4 (1998): 30–41. On Pert, see Goldberg, *Anatomy of a Scientific Discovery*, 37–41, 163–7, 197, 205; Bonnie Horrigan, 'Candace Pert, Ph.D.: Neuropeptides, AIDS, and the Science of Mind-Body Healing,' *Alternative Therapies in Health and Medicine* 1 (1995): 70–6.

115 D. Marazziti, H.S. Akiskal, A. Rossi, and G.B. Cassano, 'Alteration

of the Platelet Serotonin Transporter in Romantic Love,' *Psychological Medicine* 29 (1999): 741–5.

116 Brian Moore, *The Doctor's Wife* (New York: Farrar, Strauss, and Giroux, 1976).

117 Joan Connor, 'How to Stop Loving Someone: A Twelve-Step Program,' *TriQuarterly* 98 (winter 1996–7): 167–76.

118 Sean McArthur and Marrie Mckenna, '"Love Bug" Hits World's E-Mail,' *Globe and Mail*, 5 May 2000, A1, A11.

119 *Diagnostic and Statistical Manual of Mental Disorders: DSM-IIIR.* 3rd rev. ed. (Washington, DC: American Psychiatric Association, 1987), 199; *Diagnostic and Statistical Manual of Mental Disorders: DSM-IV,* 4th ed. (Washington, DC: American Psychiatric Association, 1994), 296–7.

120 Robert L. Spitzer et al., eds. *DSM-IV Casebook: A Learning Companion to the Diagnostic and Statistical Manual of Mental Disorders* (Washington, DC: American Psychiatric Association, 1994), 103–4.

121 Esquirol, *Mental Maladies*, 335–42. For an accessible description of this syndrome, see Rajendra D. Persaud, 'Erotomania,' *Contemporary Review* 256 (March 1990), 148–52. See also M. David Enouch and W.H. Trethown, *Uncommon Psychiatric Syndromes* (Bristol: John Wright and Sons, 1979), 15–35; Jackson, *Melancholia and Depression*, 371–2; Vladimir Lerner, Alexander Kapstan, and Eliezer Witztum, 'The Misidentification of Clerambault's and Kandinsky-Clerambault's Syndromes,' *Canadian Journal of Psychiatry* 46 (2001): 441–3.

122 Marilou McPhedran, 'The Final Report of the Task Force on Sexual Abuse of Patients' (Toronto: College of Physicians and Surgeons of Ontario, 1991); Tracey D. Smith, 'Institutionalized Violence within the Medical Profession,' in *Men and Masculinities: A Critical Anthology,* ed. Tony Haddad (Toronto: Canadian Scholars' Press, 1993), 263–75.

123 Richard D. Chessick, 'Malignant Eroticized Countertransference,' *Journal of the American Academy of Psychoanalysis* 25 (1997), 219–35; Carolyn Quadrio, 'Sex, Gender and the Impaired Therapist,' *Australian and New Zealand Journal of Psychiatry* 26 (1992): 346–63; Thomas Schill, Jeff Harsch, and Katie Ritter, 'Countertransference in the Movies: Effects on Beliefs about Psychiatric Treatment,' *Psychological Reports* 67 (1990): 399–402.

124 Duncan Spencer, *Love Gone Wrong: The Jean Harris Scarsdale Murder*

Case (New York: Signet Books, New American Library, 1981).

125 Jacques Buteau, Allain D. Lesage, and Margaret C. Kiely, 'Homicide Followed by Suicide: A Quebec Case Series, 1988–1990,' *Canadian Journal of Psychiatry* 38 (1993): 552–6; Peter M. Marzuk, Kenneth Tardiff, and Charles S. Hirsch, 'The Epidemiology of Murder-Suicide,' *JAMA* 267 (1992): 3179–83.

126 Stephan B. Hamann, Timothy D. Ely, Scott T. Grafton, and Clinton D. Kilts, 'Amygdala Activity Related to Enhanced Memory for Pleasant and Aversive Stimuli,' *Nature Neuroscience* 2 (1999): 289–93.

127 Richard D. Lane, Eric M. Reiman, Geoffrey L. Ahern, Gary E. Schwartz, and Richard J. Davidson, 'Neuroanatomical Correlates of Happiness, Sadness, and Disgust,' *American Journal of Psychiatry* 154 (1997): 926–33.

128 See, for example, Thomas E. Nordahl, Murray B. Stein, Chawki Benkelfat, William E. Semple, Paul Andreason, Zametkin Allen, Thomas W. Uhde, and Robert M. Cohen, 'Regional Cerebral Metabolic Asymmetries Replicated in an Independent Group of Patients with Panic Disorders,' *Biological Psychiatry* 44 (1998): 998–1006; Scott L. Rauch, Cary R. Savage, Nathaniel M. Alpert, Alan J. Fischman, and Michael A. Jenike, 'The Functional Neuroanatomy of Anxiety: A Study of Three Disorders Using Positron Emission Tomography and Symptom Provocation,' *Biological Psychiatry* 42 (1997): 446–52; Scott L. Rauch, Cary R. Savage, Nathaniel M. Alpert, D. Dougherty, A. Kendrick, T. Curran, H.D. Brown, P. Manzo, A.J. Fischman, and M.A. Jenike, 'Probing Striatal Function in Obsessive-Compulsive Disorder: A PET Study of Implicit Sequence Learning,' *Journal of Neuropsychiatry and Clinical Neurosciences* 9 (1997): 568–73.

129 S. Saxena, A.L. Brody, J.M. Schwartz, and L.R. Baxter Jr, 'Neuroimaging and Frontal-Subcortical Circuitry in Obsessive-Compulsive Disorder,' *British Journal of Psychiatry* 35, Supplement (1998), 26–37; S. Saxena, A.L. Brody, K.M. Maidment, J.J. Dunkin., M. Colgan, S. Alborzian, M.E. Phelps, and L.R. Baxter Jr, 'Localized Orbitofrontal and Subcortical Metabolic Changes and Predictors of Response to Paroxetine Treatment in Obsessive-Compulsive Disorder,' *Neuropsychopharmacology* 21 (1999): 683–93.

130 Elaine Hatfield and Susan Sprecher, 'Measuring Passionate Love

in Intimate Relationships,' *Journal of Adolescence* 9, no. 4 (1986): 383–410.

131 Andreas Bartels and Semir Zeki. 'The Neural Basis of Romantic Love,' *Neuroreport* 11 (2000): 3829–34.

132 Madhukar H. Trivedi, 'Functional Neuroanatomy of Obsessive-Compulsive Disorder,' *Journal of Clinical Psychiatry* 57 Supplement 8 (1996): 26–35.

133 A Canadian report on this aspect of Marazziti's research was made by Karen Birchard, 'Study Confirms That Love Can Make You Crazy,' *Medical Post* 35, 6 April 1999, 63.

134 John Harlow's report on Hazan's research originally written for the London *Sunday Times* was reprinted as front-page news in several newspapers in Canada. See, for example, John Harlow, 'Limits of Love: A Many Splendored 2 1/2 years,' *Montreal Gazette*, 25 July 1999, A1, A6; John Harlow, 'Love Is about 30 Months, Tops,' *Toronto Star*, 25 July 1999, A1.

135 Jake MacDonald, 'Doctor of Love,' *National Post*, 2 March 2002, SP1, SP6.

136 Carlo Ginzburg, 'Clues: Roots of an Evidential Paradigm [1986],' in *Clues, Myths, and the Historical Method*, trans. John and Anne Tedeschi (Baltimore and London: Johns Hopkins University Press, 1989), 96–125, esp. 124.

137 Jean-Charles Sournia, *A History of Alcoholism*, trans. Nick Hindley and Gareth Stantion (Oxford: Basil Blackwell, 1990).

138 Jeane Harper and Connie Capdevila, 'Codependency: A Critique,' *Journal of Psychoactive Drugs* 22 (1990): 285–92; Carolyn Hurcom, Alex Copello, and Jim Orford, 'The Family and Alcohol: Effects of Excessive Drinking and Conceptualizations of Spouses over Recent Decades,' *Substance Use and Misuse* 35 (2000): 473–502, esp. 486–8; J.P. Morgan, 'What Is Codependency?' *Journal of Clinical Psychology* 47 (1991): 720–9; John Steadman Rice, *A Disease of One's Own: Psychotherapy, Addiction, and the Emergence of Co–Dependency* (New Brunswick, NJ, and London: Transaction Publishers, 1996).

139 Robin Norwood, *Women Who Love Too Much: When You Keep Wishing and Hoping He'll Change* (New York: Pocket Books, 1985); Anne

Wilson Schaef, *Co-Dependence: Misunderstood – Mistreated* (Minneapolis: Winston Press, 1986).

140 *DSM-IV,* 665–6; R. Asher and D. Brissett, 'Codependency: A View from Women Married to Alcoholics,' *International Journal of Addictions* 23 (1988): 331–50; Timmen L. Cermak, 'Diagnostic Criteria for Codependency,' *Journal of Psychoactive Drugs* 18 (1986): 15–20.

141 Natasha R. Lindley, Peter J. Giordano, and Elliott D. Hammer, 'Codependency: Predictors and Psychometric Issues,' *Journal of Clinical Psychology* 55 (1999): 59–64.

142 Sally A. Farmer, 'Entitlement in Codependency: Developmental and Therapeutic Considerations,' *Journal of Addictive Diseases* 18 (1999): 55–68; H.J. Irwin, 'Codependence, Narcissism, and Childhood Trauma,' *Journal of Clinical Psychology* 51 (1995): 658–65.

143 Donna Lynn Cook and Kimberly R. Barber, 'Relationship between Social-Support, Self-Esteem, and Codependency in the African American Female,' *Journal of Cultural Diversity* 4 (1997): 32–8; H.J. Gotham and K.J. Sher, 'Do Codependent Traits Involve More Than Basic Dimensions of Personality and Psychopathology?' *Journal of Studies on Alcohol* 57 (1996): 34–9; Cyrilla Hughes-Hammer, Donna S. Martsolf, and Richard A. Zeller, 'Depression and Codependency in Women,' *Archives of Psychiatric Nursing* 12 (1998): 326–34.

144 The people of northeast Brazil have a folk disease that seems to be the mirror image of co-dependency – 'pieto aberto' (open chest). It represents the weight of having too many demands for selfless love (i.e., for husband and children); it is subversive in that it sanctions woman's fear of losing her heart to others. L.A. Rebhun, 'A Heart Too Full: The Weight of Love in Northeast Brazil,' *Journal of American Folklore* 107 (winter 1994): 167–80.

145 Páll Biering, '"Codependency": A Disease or the Root of Nursing Excellence?' *Journal of Holistic Nursing* 16 (1998): 320–37.

146 Sandra C. Anderson, 'A Critical Analysis of the Concept of Codependency,' *Social Work* 39 (1994): 677–85; S.L. Jones, 'Are We Addicted to Codependency?' *Archives of Psychiatric Nursing* 5 (1991), 55–6; Gail B. Malloy and Ann C. Berkery, 'Codependency: A Feminist Perspective,' *Journal of Psychosocial Nursing and Mental Health Services* 31 (1993): 15–19.

147 My concluding remarks have been influenced by: Ulrich Beck and
Elisabeth Beck-Gernsheim, *The Normal Chaos of Love* (Cambridge:
Polity Press, 1995); Aldo Carotenuto, *Eros and Pathos: Shades of Love
and Suffering*, trans. Charles Nopar (Toronto: Inner City Books,
1989); Cyrino, *In Pandora's Jar*; James F. Leckman and Linda C.
Mayes, 'Preoccupations and Behaviours Associated with Romantic
and Parental Love,' *Child and Adolescent Psychiatric Clinics of North
America* 8 (1999): 635–65; Rosemary Sullivan, *Labyrinth of Desire*.

148 I disagree with Celani, who contends that we are able to determine
when battered women are not really in love; however, I agree with
him on the futility of treating individual battered women when the
problem resides in society at large. David Celani, *The Illusion of
Love: Why the Battered Woman Returns to Her Abuser* (New York:
Columbia University Press, 1994), 206–9.

149 Rod Mickleburgh, 'Slash, Head Bash Normal in NHL: Player,'
Globe and Mail, 29 September 2000, A14. For another report that
mentions violence perpetrated by other sports heros, see Grant
Kerr, 'Roy Arrested after Domestic Row,' *Globe and Mail*, 23 October 2000, A1, A14.

150 Nancy Poon, 'Conceptual Issues in Defining Male Domestic Violence,' in *Men and Masculinities*, ed. Haddad, 245–61; W. Gordon
West, 'Boys, Recreation, and Violence: The Informal Education of
Some Young Canadian Males,' in ibid., 277–310. The pervasiveness
of television violence is well documented, but its negative effects
are still under dispute. See Wendy L. Josephson, *Television Violence:
A Review of the Effects on Children of Different Ages* (Ottawa: Department of Canadian Heritage and Health Canada, 1995). According
to President Bill Clinton in a 1994 speech, by age eighteen the average American will have seen 40,000 dramatized murders. Another
survey counted 1846 violent scenes in one day of television between 6 A.M. and midnight. Dave Grossman and Gloria Degaetano,
Stop Teaching Our Kids to Kill (New York: Crown Publishers, 1999),
1, 37–8.

151 Few works have explored the potential tragedy in romantic love,
which entails vulnerability and sacrifice. See especially, Sullivan
Labyrinth of Desire.

152 For a concise introduction to the rules surrounding marriage in the Catholic Church, see William H. Woestman, *Special Marriage Cases*, 3rd ed. (Bangalore: Theological Publications, 1995).

Chapter 3: Livers: The Rise of Hepatitis C

1 Hippocrates, 'Epidemics II,' section 1, chap. 10, in *Hippocrates with an English Translation*, Loeb Classical Library, vol. 7, trans. Wesley D. Smith (Cambridge, MA: Harvard University Press, 1994), 29 (leukophlegmasia).

2 Hippocrates, 'Internal Affections,' *Hippocrates with an English Translation*, Loeb Classical Library, vol. 6, ed. and trans. Paul Potter (Cambridge, MA: Harvard University Press, 1988), 70–255, esp. 164–75.

3 Aretaeus, 'Chronic Diseases, Book I, Chapter XV, "On Jaundice, or Icterus,"' in *Extant Works of Aretaeus the Cappadocian*, ed. and trans. Francis Adams (London: Sydenham Society, 1856), 324–8, esp. 327.

4 Aretaeus, 'Of Acute Diseases, Book II, Chapter VII, "On the Acute Affections about the Liver,"' in ibid., 277–9, esp. 280.

5 Aretaeus, 'Of Chronic Diseases, Book I, Chapter XIII, "On the Liver,"' in ibid., 319–22, esp. 319.

6 Aretaeus, 'Therapeutics of Acute Diseases, Book II, Chapter VI, "Cure of the Acute Affections about the Liver,"' in ibid., 440–2, esp. 440; 'On the Cure of Chronic Diseases, Book I, Chapter V "Cure of Melancholy,"' in ibid., 473–8, esp. 473.

7 Aretaeus, 'Of Chronic Diseases, Book I, Chapter XIII, "On the Liver," in ibid., 319–22, esp. 322.

8 Aretaeus, 'Chronic Diseases, Book I, Chapter XV, "On Jaundice, or Icterus,"' in ibid., 324–8, esp. 324–5. Aretaeus used the word 'viscus' for hollow as well as solid organs.

9 Ibid., 325, 327.

10 Ibid., 327–8.

11 See for example, Hippocrate, 'Des affections internes,' in *Oeuvres complètes d'Hippocrate*, vol. 7, ed. and trans. Emile Littré (Paris: Baillière, 1851), 162–303, esp. 237–43.

12 Hippocrates, 'Internal Affections,' 164–75 (passages 27, 28, 29). Celsus, *De Medicina, with an English Translation*, 3 vols., trans.

W.G. Spencer (London and Cambridge: Loeb Classical Library, Heinemann and Harvard University Press, 1960), 1: 272–3.

13 Frantisek Simon, 'Uber den Bedeutungswandel der Suffixes "-itis" und "-oma" in der medizinischen Terminologie,' *Schriftenr. Geschichte der Naturwissenschaft, Technik, und Medizin* 25 (1988): 67–83.

14 Archibaldi Pitcarnii, 'I. Elementorium medicinae,' in *Opera omnia* (Lugduni Batavorum: John Arnold Langerak, 1737), 1–183, esp. liber II, cap. 20 (on icterus and scirrhus of the the liver).

15 Jacalyn Duffin, 'Why Does Cirrhosis Belong to Laennec?' *CMAJ* 137 (1987): 393–6.

16 The first clinico-pathological description of leukemia is generally credited to Rudolf Virchow in 1847.

17 P. Stanley, 'Budd-Chiari Syndrome,' *Radiology* 170, no. 3, pt 1 (1989): 625–7.

18 For example, Gaucher's disease, a lipid-storage disorder, was first described in 1882.

19 While the symptoms provoked by parasitic infestations have been recognized since antiquity, the fields of parasitology and tropical medicine grew in the nineteenth century with the advent of medical microscopy and the identification of specific parasites. See John Farley, *Bilharzia: A History of Imperial Tropical Medicine* (Cambridge: Cambridge University Press, 1991).

20 Maxwell M. Wintrobe, ed., *Blood Pure and Eloquent: A Story of Discovery, of People, and of Ideas* (New York: McGraw-Hill, 1980).

21 Several different types of porphyria were described from the late nineteenth century into the 1960s.

22 Thalassemia or Cooley's anemia, an inherited disorder of hemoglobin production that results in liver enlargement, was first described in 1925.

23 Mirko D. Grmek, *Les maladies à l'aube de la civilisation occidentale* (Paris: Payot, 1983), 326–40.

24 M.R. Gherardini, 'Über Eine Gelbsuchtepidemie Während des Sommers 538 im Gebiet und Ancona,' *Gesnerus* 26 (1969): 145–53; A. Garcia-Kutzbach, 'Medicine among the Ancient Maya,' *Southern Medical Journal* 69 (1976): 938–40.

25 C. Chastel, 'La peste de Barcelone. Epidémie de fièvre jaune de

1821,' *Bulletin de la Société de Pathologie Exotique* 92, no. 5, pt 2 (1999), 405–7; Grmek, *Les maladies*, 29; K.D. Patterson, 'Yellow Fever Epidemics and Mortality in the United States, 1693–1905,' *Social Science and Medicine* 34 (1992), 855–65; R.L. Wilkinson, 'Yellow Fever: Ecology, Epidemiology, and Role in the Collapse of the Classic Lowland Maya Civilization,' *Medical Anthropology* 16 (1995): 269–94. Lecturing at the Collège de France in 1822 in the wake of a Barcelona epidemic, R.T.H. Laennec considered the question of 'fièvre jaune,' adopting the opinion that it was contagious. He referred also to the American experience. R.T.H. Laennec, Collège de France, 1822–23, Leçon 36, Musée Laennec, Nantes France, MS. Cl. 2 a(A), f. 14r–v.

26 Reed's priority for this observation has been challenged, but his announcement received more attention than those of his predecessors. On the modern history of yellow fever, see François Delaporte, *The History of Yellow Fever: An Essay on the Birth of Tropical Medicine* (Cambridge, MA, and London: MIT Press, 1991); Margaret Humphreys, *Yellow Fever and the South* (New Brunswick, NJ: Rutgers University Press, 1992); Miguel A. Chiong, 'Dr. Carlos Finlay and Yellow Fever,' *CMAJ* 141 (1989): 1126.

27 H.W. Baker, 'Needle Aspiration Biopsy (Hayes E. Martin),' *Ca: A Cancer Journal for Clinicians* 36 (1986): 69–70; William J. Frable, 'Fine-Needle Aspiration Biopsy: A Review,' *Human Pathology* 14 (1983): 9–28.

28 Paul B. Beeson, 'Jaundice Occurring One to Four Months after Transfusion of Blood or Plasma: Report of Seven Cases,' *JAMA* 121 (1943): 1332–4.

29 Saul Krugman, Joan Giles, and Jack Hammond, 'Infectious Hepatitis: Evidence for Two Distinctive Clinical, Epidemiological, and Immunological Types of Infection,' *JAMA* 200 (1967): 365–73; S. Krugman, 'The Willowbrook Hepatitis Studies Revisited: Ethical Aspects,' *Reviews of Infectious Diseases* 8 (1986): 157–62; Robert E. Cooke, 'Vulnerable Children,' in *Children as Research Subjects: Science, Ethics, and Law*, ed. Michael A. Grodin and Leonard H. Glantz (New York and Oxford: Oxford University Press, 1994), 193–214, esp. 201–3; Susan Lederer and Michael A. Grodin, 'Historical Overview: Pediatric Experimentation,' in ibid., 3–25, esp. 17–18.

30 See, for example, Saul Krugman being pilloried at the anti-America,

anti-racist website of 'Talking Drum: The History of Human Guinea Pigs in Amerikkka "A Few Good Mengeles,"' http://www .thetalkingdrum.com/tus2.html (accessed in 2002 and again in September 2004).

31 For an example of comparison between the two types of hepatitis, see Sheila Sherlock, *Diseases of the Liver and Biliary Tract* (Oxford: Blackwell, 1968), 320. See also Arnold R. Saslow, William M. Hammon, Russell Rule Rycheck, Eleanor Steriff, and Jessica Lewis, '"Hippie" Hepatitis: An Epidemiologic Investigation Conducted within a Population of "Street People,"' *American Journal of Epidemiology* 101 (1975): 211–19.

32 J. Garrott Allen, Donald Dawson, Wynn Seyman, and Eleanor Havens, 'Blood Transfusions and Serum Hepatitis,' *Annals of Surgery* 150 (1959): 455–68.

33 Baruch S. Blumberg, Harvey J. Alter, and Sam Visnich, 'A "New" Antigen in Leukemia Sera,' *JAMA* 191 (1965): 541–6; Alfred M. Prince, 'An Antigen Detected in the Blood during the Incubation Period of Serum Hepatitis,' *Proceedings of the National Academy of Sciences of the United States of America* 60 (1968): 814–21; Baruch S. Blumberg, B.J. Gerstley, D.A. Hungerford, W. Thomas London, and Alton I. Sutnick, 'A Serum Antigen (Australia Antigen) in Down's Syndrome, Leukemia, and Hepatitis,' *Annals of Internal Medicine* 66 (1967): 924–31.

34 Cyril Levene and Baruch S. Blumberg, 'Additional Specificities of Australia Antigen and the Possible Identification of Hepatitis Carriers,' *Nature* 221 (1969): 195–6.

35 The generous (though remunerated) contributions of hemophiliac Ted Slavin, whose blood had a high titre of hepatitis C, were lauded by the researchers at his death. Baruch S. Blumberg, Irving Millman, and W. Thomas London, 'Ted Slavin's Blood and the Development of HBV Vaccine,' *New England Journal of Medicine* 312 (1985): 189.

36 Allen et al., 'Blood Transfusions and Serum Hepatitis.'

37 Several American studies on post-transfusion hepatitis are summarized in Lewellys F. Barker and Robert J. Gerety, 'The Clinical Problem of Hepatitis Transmission,' *Progress in Clinical and Biological Research* 11 (1976): 163–82.

38 Harvey J. Alter, Paul V. Holland, Robert H. Purcell, Jerrold J.

Lander, Stephen M. Feinstone, Andrew G. Morrow, and Paul J. Schmidt, 'Posttransfusion Hepatitis after Exclusion of Commercial and Hepatitis-B Antigen-Positive Donors,' *Annals of Internal Medicine* 77 (1972): 691–9; Harvey J. Alter and Michael Houghton, 'Hepatitus C Virus and Eliminating Post-Transfusion Hepatitis,' *Nature Medicine* 6 (2000): 1082–6.

39 Alfred M. Prince, 'Can the Blood-Transmitted Hepatitis Problem Be Solved?' *Annals of the New York Academy of Sciences* 240 (1975), 191–200; J.H. Hoofnagle, R.J. Gerety, J. Thiel, and L.F. Barker, 'The Prevalence of Hepatitis B Surface Antigen in Commercially Prepared Plasma Products,' *Journal of Laboratory and Clinical Medicine* 88 (1976): 102–13.

40 Alter and Houghton, 'Hepatitus C Virus and Eliminating Post-Transfusion Hepatitis'; Barker and Gerety, 'The Clinical Problem of Hepatitis Transmission,' 177; Donald Starr, *Blood: An Epic History of Medicine and Commerce* (New York: Alfred A. Knopf, 1999), 257. The relative danger of paid donors played a key role in the successful arguments of *Gilmore v. St Anthony Hospital and the Oklahoma City Blood Bank*, which was heard in the Supreme Court of Oklahoma in 1979.

41 Currently Canada buys a portion of its fractionation products from the United States, where some donors may be paid. Also Canadian donors with special blood types are reimbursed for regular donations through pheresis.

42 Alter et al., 'Posttransfusion Hepatitis'; Sheila Sherlock, 'Hepatitis C Virus: A Historical Perspective,' *Digestive Diseases and Sciences* 41 (1996): 3S–5S.

43 Stephen M. Feinstone, Albert Z. Kapikan, and Robert H. Purcell, 'Hepatitis A: Detection by Immune Electron Microscopy of a Virus-like Antigen Associated with Acute Illness,' *Science* 182 (1973): 1026–8.

44 Stephen M. Feinstone, Albert Z. Kapikan, Robert H. Purcell, Harvey J. Alter, and Paul V. Holland, 'Transfusion-Associated Hepatitis Not Due to Viral Hepatitis Type A or B,' *New England Journal of Medicine* 292 (1975): 767–70.

45 Selma K. Dritz, 'Medical Aspects of Homosexuality,' *New England Journal of Medicine* 302 (1980): 463–4; J.L. Fluker, 'A 10-Year Study of

Homosexually Transmitted Infection,' *British Journal of Venereal Diseases* 52 (1976): 155–60; Gert G. Frösner, Holger M. Buchholz, and Hans Joachim Gerth, 'Prevalence of Hepatitis B Antibody in Prostitutes,' *American Journal of Epidemiology* 102 (1975): 241–50.

46 P. Gunby, 'Clinical Trial of Vaccine for Type B Hepatitis to Begin Next Month,' *JAMA* 241 (1979): 979–80; Dale E. Dietzman, James Harnisch, C. George Ray, E. Russell Alexander, and King K. Holmes, 'Hepatitis B Surface Antigen (HBsAg) and Antibody to HBsAg: Prevalence in Homosexual and Heterosexual Men,' *JAMA* 238 (1977): 2625–6.

47 Olaf Ringeretz and Bo Zetterberg, 'Serum Hepatitis among Swedish Track Finders,' *New England Journal of Medicine* 276 (1967): 540–6; I. Braverman, D. Wexler, and M. Oren, 'A Novel Mode of Infection with Hepatitis B: Penetrating Bone Fragments Due to the Explosion of a Suicide Bomber,' *Israel Medical Association Journal* 4 (2002): 528–9.

48 Harvey J. Alter, Paul V. Holland, Andrew G. Morrow, Robert H. Purcell, Stephen M. Feinstone, and Yasuo Moritsugu, 'Clinical and Serological Analysis of Transfusion-Associated Hepatitis,' *Lancet* 2 (1975): 838–41.

49 Jay H. Hoofnagle, Robert J. Gerety, Edward Tabor, Stephen M. Feinstone, Lewellys F. Barker, and Robert H. Purcell, 'Transmission of Non-A, Non-B Hepatitis,' *Annals of Internal Medicine* 87 (1977): 14–20; James W. Mosley, Allan G. Redeker, Stephen M. Feinstone, and Robert H. Purcell, 'Multiple Hepatitis Viruses in Multiple Attacks of Acute Viral Hepatitis,' *New England Journal of Medicine* 296 (1977): 75–8.

50 H.J. Alter, 'Transfusion Associated Non-A Non-B Hepatitis: The First Decade,' in *Viral Hepatitis and Liver Disease*, ed. A.J. Zuckerman (New York: Liss, 1988), 537–42; Alter and Houghton, 'Hepatitis C Virus and Eliminating Post-Transfusion Hepatitis'; Daniel W. Bradley, Krysztof Krawczynski, Michael J. Beach, and Michael A. Purdy, 'Non-A, Non-B Hepatitis: Toward the Discovery of Hepatitis C and E Viruses,' *Seminars in Liver Disease* 11 (1991): 128–46; Anne-Marie Couroucé, 'De l'hépatite non-A non-B à l'hépatite C,' *Transfusion Clin. Biol.* 4 (1997): 287–90; Horace Krever, *Commission of Inquiry on the Blood System in Canada, Final Report*, 3 vols (Ottawa: Canadian

Government Publishing–PWGSC, 1997), 2: 612–27; Vic Parsons, *Bad Blood: The Tragedy of the Canadian Tainted Blood Scandal* (Toronto: Lester Publishing, 1995); André Picard, *The Gift of Death: Confronting Canada's Tainted-Blood Tragedy* (Toronto: HarperCollins, 1998), 208–30; Sherlock, 'Hepatitis C Virus: A Historical Perspective'; Starr, *Blood*.

51 Hepatitis D and E were given Medical Subject Headings (MeSH) headings in 1985 and 1990, respectively. Hepatitis F and G do not yet have MeSH headings, but can be found in Medline keyword searches forward from 1994 and 1996, respectively. For accessible explanations of the newer distinctions, see Gulchin A. Ergun and Paul F. Miskovitz, 'Viral Hepatitis: The New ABC's,' *Postgraduate Medicine* 88 (1990): 69–76; D. Scott Bowden, Len D. Moaven, and Stephen A. Locarini, 'New Hepatitis Viruses: Are There Enough Letters in the Alphabet?' *Medical Journal of Australia* 164 (1996): 87–9.

52 For 1974 alone, no less than twenty review articles on the complications of using blood products are indexed in Medline. Hepatitis was the most common complication, but it was only one of several potentially fatal side effects of transfusion. See, for example, L.T. Lamont, 'Postoperative Jaundice,' *Surgical Clinics of North America* 54 (1974): 637–45.

53 Judith Graham Pool and Angela E. Shannon, 'Production of High-Potency Concentrates of Antihemophilic Globulin in a Closed-Bag System: Assay in Vitro and in Vivo,' *New England Journal of Medicine* 273 (1965): 1443–7.

54 Jane F. Desforges, 'AIDS and Preventive Treatment in Hemophilia,' *New England Journal of Medicine* 308 (1983): 94–5.

55 Christos Tsoukas, Francine Gervais, Joseph Shuster, Phil Gold, Michael O'Shaughnessy, and Marjorie Robert-Guroff, 'Association of HTLV-III Antibodies and Cellular Immune Status of Hemophiliacs,' *New England Journal of Medicine* 311 (1984): 1514–15.

56 The odds are based on the data supplied in the following: J.J. Goedert, M.G. Sarngadharan, M.E. Eyster, S.H. Weiss, A.J. Bodner, R.C. Gallo, and W.A. Blattner, 'Antibodies Reactive with Human T Cell Leukemia Viruses in the Serum of Hemophiliacs Receiving Factor VIII Concentrate,' *Blood* 65 (1985): 492–5; J.M. Soucie, R. Nuss, B. Evatt, A. Abdelhak, L. Cowan, H. Hill, M. Kolakoski, and N. Wilber,

'Mortality among Males with Hemophilia: Relations with Source of Medical Care. The Hemophilia Surveillance System Project Investigators,' *Blood* 96 (2000): 437–42.; I.R. Walker and J.A. Julian, 'Causes of Death in Canadians with Haemophilia 1980–1995. Association of Hemophilia Clinic Directors of Canada,' *Haemophilia* 4 (1998): 714–20; World Hemophilia Federation, *Report on the Global Survey 2001* (Montreal, 2001); T.T. Yee, A. Griffioen, C.A. Sabin, G. Dusheiko, and C.A. Lee, 'The Natural History of HCV in a Cohort of Haemophilic Patients Infected between 1961 and 1985,' *Gut* 47 (2000): 845–51.

57 A 1975 study showed that 40 per cent of factor IX concentrates were contaminated with hepatitis B and that this virus represented only a quarter of the post-transfusion hepatitis. Hoofnagle et al., 'The Prevalence of Hepatitis B Surface Antigen.'

58 Mirko D. Grmek, *History of AIDS*, trans. Russell C. Maulitz and Jacalyn Duffin (Princeton, NJ: Princeton University Press, 1990).

59 Krever, *Commission of Inquiry*, 3: 952.

60 Ibid.

61 Starr, *Blood*, 319; Alter and Houghton, 'Hepatitis C Virus and Eliminating Posttransfusion Hepatitis.'

62 Krever, *Commission of Inquiry*, 1: xxii–xxv. R.S. Remis, M.V. O'Shaughnessy, C. Tsoukas, G.H. Growe, M.T. Schechter, R.W. Palmer, and D.N. Lawrence, 'HIV Transmission to Patients with Hemophilia by Heat-Treated, Donor-Screened Factor Concentrate,' *CMAJ* 142 (1990): 1247–54.

63 Harvey J. Alter, Betsy W. Jett, Alan J. Polito, Patrizia Farci, Jacqueline C. Melpolder, James W. Shih, Yohko Shimizu, and Robert H. Purcell, 'Analysis of the Role of Hepatitis C in Transfusion-Associated Hepatitis,' in *Viral Hepatitis and Liver Disase*, ed. F. Blaine Hollinger, Stanley M. Lemon, and Harold Margolis (Baltimore: Williams and Wilkins, 1991), 396–402; Couroucé, 'De l'hépatite non-A non-B'; A. Giulivi, M.T. Aye, E. Gray, V. Scalia, P. Gill, and G. Cheng, 'Anti-Hepatitis C Virus (HCV) Screening at a Canadian Red Cross Center: Significance of a Positive c100 HCV Enzyme-Linked Immunosorbent Assay,' *Transfusion* 32 (1992): 309–11.

64 S.V. Feinman, B. Berris, and S. Bojarski, 'Postransfusion Hepatitis in Toronto, Canada,' *Gastroenterology* 95 (1988), 464–9; M.A. Blajchman,

S.V. Feinman, and S.B. Bull, 'The Incidence of Post-Transfusion Hepatitis,' *New England Journal of Medicine* 328 (1993): 1280–1.

65 See, for example, Krever, *Commission of Inquiry*, 1: xxix–xxx.

66 D.W. Bradley, E.H. Cook, J.E. Maynard, K.A. McCaustland, J.W. Ebert, G.H. Dolana, R.A. Petzel, R.J. Kantor, A. Heilbrunn, H.A. Fields, and B.L Murphy, 'Experimental Infection of Chimpanzees with Antihemophilic (Factor VIII) Materials: Recovery of Virus-Like Particles Associated with Non-A, Non-B Hepatitis,' *Journal of Medical Virology* 3 (1979): 253–69; D.W. Bradley, 'Studies of Non-A, Non-B Hepatitis and Characterization of the Hepatitis C Virus in Chimpanzees,' *Current Topics in Microbiology and Immunology* 242 (2000): 1–23.

67 Koch's postulates are a set of four logical conditions that must be filled before an infectious agent can be established as the cause of a disease. They are named for the German scientist Robert Koch, who used these postulates to prove that tuberculosis was caused by a specific bacterium. See K. Codell Carter, *The Rise of Causal Concepts of Disease: Case Histories* (Aldershot: Ashgate, 2003), 129–45, 196–9.

68 Alter and Houghton, 'Hepatitis C Virus and Eliminating Posttransfusion Hepatitis.'

69 D.W. Bradley, J.E. Maynard, H. Popper, J.W. Ebert, E.H. Cook, H.A. Fields, and B.J. Kemler, 'Persistent Non-A, Non-B Hepatitis in Experimentally Infected Chimpanzees,' *Journal of Infectious Diseases* 143 (1981): 210–18; N. Simon, J.P. Mery, C. Trepo, L. Vitvitski, and A. M. Couroucé, 'A Non-A Non-B Hepatitis Epidemic in a HB Antigen-Free Haemodialysis Unit: Demonstration of Serological Markers of Non-A Non-B Virus,' *Proceedings of the European Dialysis and Transplant Association* 17 (1980): 173–8.

70 This early article recommended the use of another liver enzyme, the SGOT. Nils Bang, Paul Ruegsegger, Allyn B. Ley, and John S. LaDue, 'Detection of Hepatitis Carriers by Serum Glutamic Oxalacetic Transaminase,' *JAMA* 171 (1959): 2303–6; Prince, 'Can the Blood-Transmitted Hepatitis Problem Be Solved?'

71 For a more general discussion of the problem caused by the current scientific preference for single disease entities and single causes, see Charles E. Rosenberg, 'The Tyranny of Diagnosis: Specific Entities and Individual Experience,' *Milbank Quarterly* 80 (2002): 237–60.

72 Harvey J. Alter, Robert H. Purcell, P.V. Holland, D.W. Alling, and D.E. Koziol, 'Donor Transaminase and Recipient Hepatitis. Impact on Blood Transfusion Services,' *JAMA* 246 (1981): 630–4.

73 C.E. Stevens, R.D. Aach, F.B. Hollinger, J.W. Mosley, W. Szmuness, R. Kahn, J. Werch, and V. Edwards, 'Hepatitis B Virus Antibody in Blood Donors and the Occurrence of Non-A, Non-B Hepatitis in Transfusion Recipients: An Analysis of the Transfusion-Transmitted Viruses Study,' *Annals of Internal Medicine* 101 (1984): 733–8; D.E. Koziol, P.V. Holland, D.W. Alling, J.C. Melpolder, R.E. Solomon, R.H. Purcell, L.M. Hudson, F.J. Shoup, H. Krakauer, and H.J. Alter, 'Antibody to Hepatitis B Core Antigen as a Paradoxical Marker for Non-A, Non-B Hepatitis Agents in Donated Blood,' *Annals of Internal Medicine* 104 (1986): 488–95.

74 Marc D. Silverstein, Albert G. Mulley, and Jules L. Dienstag, 'Should Donor Blood Be Screened for Elevated Alanine Aminotransferase Levels? A Cost-Effectiveness Analysis,' *JAMA* 252 (1984): 2839–45.

75 Leonard B. Seeff and Jules L. Dienstag, 'Transfusion-Associated Non-A, Non-B Hepatitis: Where Do We Go from Here?' *Gastroenterology* 95 (1988): 530–3.

76 Ibid. For a general discussion of these thorny matters, see Rosenberg, 'The Tyranny of Diagnosis,'

77 Krever, *Commission of Inquiry*, 2: 659–86; Blajchman et al., 'The Incidence of Post-Transfusion Hepatitis'; M.A. Blajchman, S.B. Bull, and S.V. Feinman, 'Post Transfusion Hepatitis: Impact of Non-A, Non-B Surrogate Tests. Canadian Post-Transfusion Hepatitis Prevention Study,' *Lancet* 345 (1995): 21–5.

78 Picard, *Gift of Death*, 215–20.

79 Qui Lim Choo, George Kuo, Amy J. Weiner, Lacy R. Overby, Daniel W. Bradley, and Michael Houghton, 'Isolation of a cDNA Clone Derived from a Blood-Borne Non-A Non-B Viral Hepatitis Genome,' *Science* 244 (1989): 359–61.

80 G. Kuo, Q.L. Choo, H.J. Alter, G.L. Gitnick, A.G. Redeker, R.H. Purcell, T. Miyamura, J.L. Dienstag, M.J. Alter, C.E. Stevens, 'An Assay for Circulating Antibodies to a Major Etiologic Virus of Human Non-A, Non-B Hepatitis,' *Science* 244 (1989): 362–4; H.J. Alter, R.H. Purcell, J.W. Shih, J.C. Melpolder, M. Houghton, Q.L. Choo, and G. Kuo,

'Detection of Antibody to Hepatitis C Virus in Prospectively Followed Transfusion Recipients with Acute and Chronic Non-A, Non-B Hepatitis,' *New England Journal of Medicine* 321 (1989): 1494–500.

81 Alter, 'Transfusion Associated Non-A Non-B Hepatitis: The First Decade'; Harvey J. Alter and Alfred M. Prince, 'Transfusion-Associated Non-A, Non-B Hepatitis: An Assessment of the Causative Agent and Its Clinical Impact,' *Transfusion Medicine Reviews* 2 (1988): 288–93.

82 Harvey J. Alter, 'Descartes before the Horse: I Clone, therefore I Am: The Hepatitis C Virus in Current Perspective,' *Annals of Internal Medicine* 115 (1991): 644–9.

83 Alter and Houghton, 'Hepatitus C Virus and Eliminating Post-Transfusion Hepatitis'; R. De Vos et al., 'Ultrastructural Visualization of Hepatitis C Virus Components in Human and Primate Liver Biopsies,' *Journal of Hepatology* 37 (2002): 370–9.

84 Krever, *Commission of Inquiry*, 1: xxxi.

85 Alter and Houghton, 'Hepatitus C Virus and Eliminating Post-Transfusion Hepatitis.' Younger readers may not be familiar with this phrase from a toothpaste commercial in the 1960s.

86 Krever, *Commission of Inquiry*, 1: xxxi; 2: 668–73; Morris Blajchman, interview, 20 December 2002.

87 Blajchman et al., 'The Incidence of Post-Transfusion Hepatitis.'

88 Blajchman et al., 'Post Transfusion Hepatitis: Impact of Non-A, Non-B Surrogate Tests.'

89 Morris Blajchman, interview, 20 December 2002.

90 In early September 1993, as the Blajchman–Feinman results were being released, the *Globe and Mail* ran a series of front-page articles on the issue of blood safety in which the major focus was HIV. See André Picard, 'Restoring Faith in the Safety Net. Blood Test, Part 1,' *Globe and Mail*, 4 September 1993, A1, A6; 'Family Fights to Ensure Pain Not in Vain. Blood Test, Part 2,' *Globe and Mail*, 6 September 1993, A1, A4; 'France Makes Example of Misdeeds. Blood Test, Part 3,' *Globe and Mail*, 7 September 1993, A1, A4; 'Lending an Arm to Save Lives, Money. Blood Test, Part 4,' *Globe and Mail*, 8 September 1993, A1, A6.

91 I am grateful to my colleague Patricia Peppin of Queen's University Faculty of Law for bringing this collection of cases to my attention.

92 Contrast the decision in *Hegarty v. Shine* (1878) in Ireland High
   Court of Justice, *Cox's Criminal Cases*, vol. XIV, 1877–82, 124–35 and
   145–52, with the decision rendered in Canada 120 years later in
   Regina v. Cuerrier, [1998] 2 S.C.R., 371–441. On this point see Philip
   H. Osborne, *Law of Torts* (Toronto: Irwin Law, 1999), 244–5. I am
   grateful to Horace Krever for bringing these fascinating cases to
   my attention.

93 Starr, *Blood*, 330–4; P. Aldhous and C. Tastemain, 'Three Physicians
   Convicted in French "Blood-Supply Trial,"' *Science* 258 (1992): 735;
   Declan Butler, 'Verdict in French Blood Trial Shames Science,'
   Nature 359 (1992): 764.

94 J.P. Allain, 'French Blood Contamination,' *Nature* 360 (1992): 99.

95 Krever, *Commission of Inquiry*, 3: 1033–4; Keither Wilson, 'Ireland
   Announces Compensation for Hepatitis C,' *British Medical Journal*
   311 (1995): 771.

96 The names of the applicants and the details of their complaint can
   be read at the website of the Canadian Legal Information Institute,
   Attorney General of Canada v. Horace Krever (1996–06–27), FC T-154-
   96, http://www.canlii.org/ca/cas/fct/1996/1996fct10032.html
   (accessed February 2005).

97 Picard, *Gift of Death*, 218.

98 Wayne Kondro, 'Revelations Rock Canada's Tainted-Blood
   Inquiry,' *Lancet* 347 (1996): 1178; David Spurgeon, 'Canada's HIV
   Blood Inquiry Turns Poisonous,' *Nature* 384 (1997): 602.

99 David Spurgeon, 'Canadian Inquiry Calls for "Safety First" Blood
   Agency,' *Nature* 390 (1997): 432.

100 Krever, *Commission of Inquiry*. For more on the political aspects of
    the history of blood services in Canada, see Adam D. McDonald,
    'Collaboration, Competition and Coercion: Canadian Federalism
    and Blood System Governance' (MA thesis, University of Water-
    loo, Waterloo, Ontario, 2004).

101 Krever, *Commission of Inquiry*, 2: 707.

102 Morris Blajchman, interview, 20 December 2002. The media, which
    had not been present at the testimony, later claimed that Blajch-
    man's tears were the result of lawyers' questioning over mistakes
    in the past. Canadian Press Newswire, 'Red Cross Centre Sent out
    Possibly Deadly Blood While It Had Safe Blood,' 21 October 1994.

103 Morris A. Blajchman and Harvey G. Klein, 'Looking Back in Anger,' *Transfusion Medicine Reviews* 11 (1997): 1–5; Anne Mullens, 'Concern Mounts as Transfusion Medicine Loses Its Lustre,' *CMAJ* 158 (1998): 1499–502; Morris Blajchman, interview, 23 October 2002.

104 Retired anesthetist Ray Matthews, a former chairman of the Blood Tranfusion Service (BTS) Advisory Committee, wrote to me: 'During the Krever study no Chairman of the BTS Advisory Committee was called to testify. (There were three during this period, myself, John Bienenstock, Blair Whittemore.) We were scheduled but for reasons unknown were cancelled. Scientific questions were inappropriately directed to some lay Red Cross board members. Naturally they were unable to answer intelligently and I believe were unnecessarily embarrassed along with the Canadian Red Cross' (undated personal communication, spring 2003).

105 The Royal Canadian Mounted Police immediately began investigations. Not until five years later (and a month after this lecture was read), were the first charges laid against four individuals involved with the administration of the old blood system. André Picard, 'RCMP Lay 32 Charges in Tainted-Blood Case,' *Globe and Mail*, 21 November 2002, A1, A6.

106 Four years later, the new Canadian Blood Service still experiences growing pains. Haunted by the collapse of its predecessor, it has tried to avoid the same mistakes by sending out communiqués and hosting conferences. Nevertheless, a review completed in 2001 by a three-person task force, made up of William Leiss, Hugh Segal, and Timothy Plumptre, suggested that it could do more to avoid secrecy. Perhaps in response to this criticism and in the wake of the 11 September 2001 tragedy, the director, Dr Graham Sher, announced a possible threat of terrorist attacks on the blood supply, admitting that 'there is no immediate use the public can make of the warning.' John Saunders, 'Letter Threatens Canada's Blood System,' *Globe and Mail*, 7 November 2001, A9.

107 Krever, *Commission of Inquiry*, 3: 1045.

108 Ibid., 1034.

109 Ibid., 1045.

110 Ibid., 1029–45.

111 The law-medicine analogy is mine, but it was inspired by Rosenberg, 'The Tyranny of Diagnosis.'

112 D. Spurgeon, 'Canadians Sue over Hepatitis C Infection,' *British Medical Journal* 315 (1997): 330.

113 Figure 3.4 is based on annual reports in the *Canada Communicable Disease Reports*. On the emergence of hepatitis C as a political issue, see Michael Orsini, 'The Politics of Naming, Blaming, and Claiming: HIV, Hepatitis C, and the Emergence of Blood Activism in Canada,' *Canadian Journal of Political Science / Revue Canadien de Science Politique* 35 (2002): 475–98.

114 André Picard, 'Hepatitis C Victims Get Little of Fund,' *Globe and Mail*, 1 April 2002, A1, A7.

115 'Seeing Red [photo: death's head protestor],' *Kingston Whig-Standard*, 21 September 2000, 14; Kim Lunman, 'Liver Transplant Hopes Rest on Prayer,' *Globe and Mail*, 4 November 2000, A4.

116 Wayne Kondro, 'Canada's Hepatitis C Compensation Derailed,' *Lancet* 351 (1998): 1415; 'Judge Approves Hepatitis C Settlement,' *Globe and Mail*, 27 June 2001, A7. At the time of writing, pressure to reopen the package continues.

117 Victor Blanchette, Irwin Walker, Peter Gill, Margaret Adams, Robin Roberts, and Martin Inwood, 'Hepatitis C Infection in Patients with Hemophilia: Results of a National Survey. Canadian Hemophilia Clinic Directors Group,' *Transfusion Medicine Reviews* 8 (1994): 210–17.

118 See the website http://www.hemophilia.ca/. See also Wayne Kondro, 'Compensation for Canada's Hepatitis C Victims to Be Re-evaluated,' *Lancet* 351 (1998): 1567; Wayne Kondro, 'Revised Estimates of Hepatitis C from Tainted Blood Published,' *Lancet* 352 (1998): 466.

119 For higher estimates, see Shimian Zou, Martin Tepper, and Antonio Giulivi, 'Current Status of Hepatitis C in Canada,' *Canadian Journal of Public Health* 91, Supplement 1 (2000): S4–S9.

120 Wayne Kondro, 'Revelations Rock Canada's Tainted-Blood Inquiry.'

121 In February 1992, Italy implemented monthly pensions for life on a sliding scale related to the severity of the illness. Krever, *Commission of Inquiry*, 3: 1033.

122 Anonymous, 'The National Institutes of Health Consensus Development Conference: Management of Hepatitis C, Bethesda MD, 24 to 26 March 1997,' *Hepatology* 26, no. 3, Supplement 1 (1997): 1S–156S; Susannah Benady, 'Alcohol a Major Predictor of Hepatitis C Recovery,' *Medical Post* 15 May 2001, 7; Christian Trépo and Rafael Esteban, 'Chronic HCV Infection; Public Health Threat and Emerging Consensus, Conference held in Vienna Austria, 27 to 28 October 1995,' *Digestive Diseases and Sciences* 41, no. 12, Supplement (1996): 1S–135S.

123 Callum et al., 'An Evaluation of the Process and Costs.'

124 Jeannie L. Callum, Peter H. Pinkerton, Ahmed S. Coovadia, Anne E. Thomson, and Frankie Dewsbury, 'An Evaluation of the Process and Costs Associated with Targeted Lookbacks for HCV and General Notification of Transfusion Recipients,' *Transfusion* 40 (2000): 1169–75; Mindy Goldman and Anne Long, 'Hepatitis C Lookback in Canada,' *Vox Sanguinis* 78, Supplement 2 (2000): 249–52; Mindy Goldman and Gwendoline Spurll, 'Hepatitis C Lookback,' *Current Opinion in Hematology* 7 (2000): 392–6; Nancy Heddle, John G. Kelton, Fiona Smaill, Krista Foss, Jennifer Everson, Cynthia Janzen, Chris Walker, Marak Jones, and Debby Hammons, 'A Canadian Hospital-Based HIV/Hepatitis Look-Back Notification Program,' *CMAJ* 157 (1997): 149–54; J.M. Langley, S.G. Squires, D.M. MacDonald, D. Anderson, K. Peltekian, and J.W. Scott, 'Evaluation of the Notification of Hepatitis C Risk to Children Who Received Unscreened Blood or Blood Products,' *Communicable Disease and Public Health* 4 (2001): 288–92; A. Long, G. Spurll, H. Demers, and M. Goldman, 'Targeted Hepatitis C Lookback: Quebec, Canada,' *Transfusion* 39 (1999): 194–200; E.A. Roberts, S.M. King, M. Fearon, and N. McGee, 'Hepatitis C in Children after Transfusion: Assessment by Look Back Studies,' *Acta Gastroenterologica Belgica* 61 (1998): 195–7.

125 Statistics last revised October 2000 from factsheet at the World Health Organization website, http://www.who.int/mediacentre/factsheets/fs164/en (accessed December 2002 and September 2004). See also Anonymous, 'Hepatitis C: Needles and Haystacks,' *The Economist*, 1 November 2003, 75; Benady, 'Alcohol a Major Predictor'; Harvey J. Alter and Leonard B. Seeff, 'Recovery, Persis-

tence, and Sequelae in Hepatitis C Virus Infection: A Perspective on Long-Term Outcome,' *Seminars in Liver Disease* 20 (2000): 17–35; T. Jake Liang, Barbara Rehermann, Leonard B. Seeff, and Jay H. Hoofnagle, 'Pathogenesis, Natural History, Treatment, and Prevention of Hepatitis C,' *Annals of Internal Medicine* 132 (2000): 296–305; Leonard B. Seeff, 'The Natural History of Hepatitis C: A Quandary,' *Hepatology* 28 (1997): 1710–12; Leonard B. Seeff, 'Natural History of Hepatitis C,' *American Journal of Medicine* 107, no. 6B (1999): 10S–15S.

126 J.B. Epstein, G. Rea, C.H. Sherlock, and R.G. Mathias, 'Continuing Investigation and Controversy Regarding Risk of Transmission of Infection via Dental Handpieces,' *Journal of the Canadian Dental Association* 62 (1996): 485–91; C.J. Tibbs, 'Methods of Transmission of Hepatitis C,' *Journal of Viral Hepatitis* 2 (1995): 113–19.

127 Seeff, 'Natural History of Hepatitis C.'

128 Benady, 'Alcohol a Major Predictor.'

129 Statistics from the website of the U.S. Centers for Disease Control, Hepatitis C factsheet, updated August 2004: http://www.cdc .gov/ncidod/diseases/hepatitis/c/fact.htm (accessed September 2004).

130 Alter and Houghton, 'Hepatitus C Virus and Eliminating Post-Transfusion Hepatitis'; Anonymous 'Needles and Haystacks'; Anonymous, 'Blood Transfusion: Cleaning Up,' *The Economist*, 14 June 2003, 80.

131 H. Alter, cited in Benady, 'Alcohol a Major Predictor.' See also A.I. Sharara, 'Chronic Hepatitis C,' *Southern Medical Journal* 90 (1997): 872–7.

132 See, for example, A. Andonov and R.K. Chaudhury, 'Genotyping of Canadian Hepatitis C Virus Isolates by PCR,' *Journal of Clinical Microbiology* 32 (1994): 2031–4; P. Chauveau, 'Epidemiology of Hepatitis C Virus Infection in Chronic Hemodialysis,' *Nephrology, Dialysis, Transplantation* 11, Supplement 4 (1996): 39–41; Jérôme Gournay, Patrick Marcellin, Michèle Martinot-Peignoux, Claude Degott, Franck Gabriel, Françoise Courtois, Michel Branger, Anne Marie Wild, Serge Erlinger, and Jean-Pierre Benhamou, 'Hepatitis C Genotypes in French Blood Donors,' *Journal of Medical Virology* 45 (1995): 399–404.

133 Elizabeth Stratton, Lamont Sweet, Arleen Latorrca-Walsh, and Paul R. Gully, 'Hepatitis C in Prince Edward Island: A Descriptive Review of Reported Cases, 1990–1995,' *Canadian Journal of Public Health* 88 (1997): 91–4.

134 J. Sandhu, J.K. Preiksaitis, P.M. Campbell, K.C. Carrière, and P.A. Hessel, 'Hepatitis C: Prevalence and Risk Factors in the Northern Alberta Dialysis Population,' *American Journal of Epidemiology* 150 (1999): 58–66.

135 D.B. Smith and P. Simmonds, 'Review: Molecular Epidemiology of Hepatitis C Virus,' *Journal of Gastroenterology and Hepatology* 12 (1997): 522–7.

136 Leonard B. Seeff, Richard N. Miller, Charles S. Rabkin, Zelma Bushell-Bales, Kelle D. Straley-Eeson, Bonnie L. Smoack, Lelye D. Johnson, Stephen R. Lee, and Edward L. Kaplan, '45-Year Follow-up of Hepatitis C Virus Infection in Healthy Young Adults,' *Annals of Internal Medicine* 132 (2000): 105–11. See also this Internet report about Seeff's work: Jamie Talan, '1948 GIs Key to Hepatitis C / Study Wants to Know Effect on Their Health, 05-21-1999,' A24, http://hepatitis-central.com/hcv/vets/1948.html (accessed September 2004).

137 Picard, 'Hepatitis C Victims Get Little of Fund.'

138 Rob Guild, 'Hep C Victim Fights for Compensation: Man Denied Money over Adolescent Indiscretion with Intravenous Drug,' *Toronto Star*, 13 December 1999, A6.

139 Heddle et al., 'A Canadian Hospital-Based HIV/Hepatitis Look-Back Notification Program.'

140 Roberts et al., 'Hepatitis C in Children.'

141 Survival after transfusion varies greatly depending on the underlying cause. For example, one study showed two-year survival rates after massive transfusion to be 100 per cent for obstetrical bleeding and 38 per cent for bleeding associated with liver failure. P.R. Sawyer and C.R. Harrison. 'Massive Transfusion in Adults: Diagnoses, Survival, and Blood Bank Support,' *Vox Sanguinis* 58 (1990): 199–203

142 C. Botté and C. Janot, 'Epidemiology of HCV Infection in the General Population and in Blood Transfusion,' *Nephrology Dialysis Transplantation* 11, Supplement 4 (1996): 19–21; Annemarie Wasley

and Miriam J. Alter, 'Epidemiology of Hepatitis C: Geographic Differences and Temporal Trends,' *Seminars in Liver Disease* 20 (2000): 1–16.

143 David M. Patrick, Jane A. Buxton, Mark Bigham, and Richard G. Mathias, 'Public Health and Hepatitis C,' *Canadian Journal of Public Health* 91, Supplement 1 (2000): S18–21; David M. Patrick, Mark W. Tyndall, Peter G. Cornelisse, Kathy Li, Chris H. Sherlock, Michael L. Rekart, Steffanie A. Strathdee, Sue L. Currie, Martin T. Schechter, and Michael V. O'Shaughnessy, 'Incidence of Hepatitis C Virus Infection among Injection Drug Users during an Outbreak of HIV Infection,' *CMAJ* 165 (2001): 889–95.

144 Sandhu et al., 'Hepatitis C: Prevalence and Risk Factors'; Sharara, 'Chronic Hepatitis C'; Tibbs, 'Methods of Transmission of Hepatitis C'; Takeshi Utsumi, Etsuo Hashimoto, Yusuke Okumura, Makiko Takananagi, Hiroaki Nishikawa, Mika Kigawa, Nobuchio Kumakura, and Hiroyuko Toyokawa, 'Heterosexual Activity as a Risk Factor for the Transmission of Hepatitis C Virus,' *Journal of Medical Virology* 46, no. 2 (1995): 122–5; Wasley and Alter, 'Epidemiology of Hepatitis C.'

145 Anonymous, 'Ex-star of Baywatch Has Contracted Hepatitis C,' *Globe and Mail*, 21 March 2002, A15. More information appeared temporarily at the *Globe* website than in the printed paper.

146 Studies in two of Kingston's federal prisons found HCV seropositivity in nearly 40 per cent of inmates be they male or female. P.M. Ford, C. White, H. Kaufmann, J. MacTavish, M. Pearson, S. Ford, P.S. Mistry, and P. Connop, 'Voluntary Screening for Hepatitis C in a Canadian Federal Penitentiary for Men,' *Canada Communicable Disease Report* 21 (1995): 134–5; Peter M. Ford, Cheryl White, Hannah Kaufmann, J. MacTavish, Mary Pearson, Sally Ford, Perin Sankar-Mistry, and Peter Connop, 'Voluntary Anonymous Linked Study of the Prevalence of HIV Infection and Hepatitis C among Inmates in a Canadian Federal Penitentiary for Women,' *CMAJ* 153 (1995): 1605–9.

147 Hieronymus David Gaubius, *Institutiones pathologiae medicinalis* (Lipsiae: Joannis Pauli Krausii Bibliopolae Viennensis, 1759), 278 (article #542).

148 A letter sent by a hemophiliac to the premier of his province and

cited by Krever emphasizes strain on lovers in the context of this illness. The writer describes what it is like 'to lie beside the woman you love for five years and be mortally afraid to touch her.' After describing his divorce, he closed with these words: '[t]he irony of this situation is, when we desperately need ... a loving relationship to fight the stress of AIDS – we are denied it.' Krever, *Commission of Inquiry*, 2: 718.

149 I have not uncovered the logic that justified less compensation to the sexual partners of people who became HIV-positive from blood transfusion. Perhaps the assumption is that engaging in sex somehow makes the spouse culpable and lessens the onus on society. For details on the package, see Wayne Kondro, 'Curtailed Canadian HIV Compensation,' *Lancet* 343 (1994): 783–4.

150 Roberts et al., 'Hepatitis C in Children'; Wasley and Alter, 'Epidemiology of Hepatitis C'; Zou, Tepper, and Giulivi, 'Current Status of Hepatitis C in Canada.'

151 D. Bresters, E.P. Mauser-Bunschoten, H.W. Reesink, G. Roosendaal, C.L. van der Poel, R.A. Chamuleau, P.L.M. Jansen, C.J. Weegink, H.T.M. Cuypers, P.N. Lelie, and H.M. Van de Berg, 'Sexual Transmission of Hepatitis C Virus,' *Lancet* 342 (1993): 210–11; Cees L. van der Poel, H. Theo Cuyper, and Henk W. Reesink, 'Hepatitis C Six Years On,' *Lancet* 344 (1994): 1475–9; Stuart C. Gordon, Ashe H. Patel, Gregory W. Kulkesza, Robert Barnes, and Ann L. Silverman, 'Lack of Evidence for the Heterosexual Transmission of Hepatitis C,' *American Journal of Gastroenterology* 87 (1992): 1849–51.

152 Yosihiro Akahane, M. Kojima, Y. Sugai, M. Sakamoto, Y. Miyazaki, T. Tanaka, F. Tsuda, S. Mishiro, H. Okamoto, and Y. Miyakawa, 'Hepatitis C Virus Infection in Spouses of Patients with Type C Chronic Liver Disease,' *Annals of Internal Medicine* 115 (1994): 748–52; M. Elaine Eyster, Harvey J. Alter, Louis M. Aledort, Stella Quan, Angelos Hatzakis, and James J. Goedert, 'Heterosexual Co-Transmission of Hepatitis C Virus (HCV) and Human Immunodeficiency Virus (HIV),' *Annals of Internal Medicine* 115 (1991): 764–8.

153 Anonymous, 'Reported Cases of Hepatitis A, B, and C in Canada – 1990–1999,' *Canada Communicable Disease Report* 20, Supplement (2001): 24–5, 56–7, 110–11.

154 U.S. Centers for Disease Control, 'Recommendations for Prevention and Control of Hepatitis C Virus (HCV) Infection and HCV-Related Chronic Disease,' *Morbidity and Mortality Weekly Reports* 47 (RR–19) (1998): 1–38.
155 Viral Hepatitis C Factsheet, http://www.cdc.gov/ncidod/ diseases/hepatitis/c/fact.htm (accessed September 2004).

Bibliography

Ackerman, Diane. *A Natural History of Love* (New York: Vintage Books, 1994.

Akahane, Yosihiro, M. Kojima, Y. Sugai, M. Sakamoto, Y. Miyazaki, T. Tanaka, F. Tsuda, S. Mishiro, H. Okamoto, and Y. Miyakawa. 'Hepatitis C Virus Infection in Spouses of Patients with Type C Chronic Liver Disease.' *Annals of Internal Medicine* 115 (1994): 748–52.

Aldhous, P., and C. Tastemain. 'Three Physicians Convicted in French "Blood-Supply Trial."' *Science* 258 (1992): 735.

Allain, J.P. 'French Blood Contamination.' *Nature* 360 (1992): 99.

Allen, J. Garrott, Donald Dawson, Wynn Seyman, and Eleanor Havens. 'Blood Transfusions and Serum Hepatitis.' *Annals of Surgery* 150 (1959): 455–68.

Allen, Peter Lewis. *The Wages of Sin: Sex and Disease, Past and Present.* Chicago: University of Chicago Press, 2000.

Alter, Harvey J. 'Descartes before the Horse: I Clone, therefore I Am: The Hepatitis C Virus in Current Perspective.' *Annals of Internal Medicine* 115 (1991): 644–9.

– 'Transfusion Associated Non-A Non-B Hepatitis: The First Decade.' In *Viral Hepatitis and Liver Disease*, ed. A.J. Zuckerman, 537–42. New York: Liss, 1988.

Alter, Harvey J., Paul V. Holland, Andrew G. Morrow, Robert H. Purcell, Stephen M. Feinstone, and Yasuo Moritsugu. 'Clinical and Serological Analysis of Transfusion-Associated Hepatitis.' *Lancet* 2 (1975): 838–41.

Alter, Harvey J., Paul V. Holland, Robert H. Purcell, Jerrold J. Lander, Stephen M. Feinstone, Andrew G. Morrow, and Paul J. Schmidt. 'Posttransfusion Hepatitis after Exclusion of Commercial and Hepatitis-B Antigen-Positive donors.' *Annals of Internal Medicine* 77 (1972): 691–9.

Alter, Harvey J., and Michael Houghton. 'Hepatitus C Virus and Eliminating Post-Transfusion Hepatitis.' *Nature Medicine* 6 (2000): 1082–6.

Alter, Harvey J., Betsy W. Jett, Alan J. Polito, Patrizia Farci, Jacqueline C. Melpolder, James W. Shih, Yohko Shimizu, and Robert H. Purcell. 'Analysis of the Role of Hepatitis C in Transfusion-Associated Hepatitis.' In *Viral Hepatitis and Liver Disase*, ed. F. Blaine Hollinger, Stanley M. Lemon, and Harold Margolis, 396–402. Baltimore: Williams and Wilkins, 1991.

Alter, Harvey J., and Alfred M. Prince. 'Transfusion-Associated Non-A, Non-B Hepatitis: An Assessment of the Causative Agent and Its Clinical Impact.' *Transfusion Medicine Reviews* 2 (1988): 288–93.

Alter, Harvey J., Robert H. Purcell, P.V. Holland, D.W. Alling, and D.E. Koziol. 'Donor Transaminase and Recipient Hepatitis. Impact on Blood Transfusion Services.' *JAMA* 246 (1981): 630–4.

Alter, Harvey J., R.H. Purcell, J.W. Shih, J.C. Melpolder, M. Houghton, Q.L. Choo, and G. Kuo. 'Detection of Antibody to Hepatitis C Virus in Prospectively followed Transfusion Recipients with Acute and Chronic Non-A, Non-B Hepatitis.' *New England Journal of Medicine* 321 (1989): 1494–500.

Alter, Harvey J., and Leonard B. Seeff. 'Recovery, Persistence, and Sequelae in Hepatitis C Virus Infection: A Perspective on Long-Term Outcome.' *Seminars in Liver Disease* 20 (2000): 17–35.

Amundsen, Darryl W. 'Romanticizing the Ancient Medical Profession.' *Bulletin of the History of Medicine* 48 (1974): 328–37.

Anderson, Sandra C. 'A Critical Analysis of the Concept of Codependency.' *Social Work* 39 (1994): 677–85.

Andonov A., and R.K. Chaudhury. 'Genotyping of Canadian Hepatitis C Virus Isolates by PCR.' *Journal of Clinical Microbiology* 32 (1994): 2031–4.

Andreas Capellanus. *De amore. Andreas Capellanus on Love*, ed. G. Walsh. Worcester and London: Trinity Press, 1982.

Anonymous. 'Blood Transfusion: Cleaning Up.' *The Economist*, 14 June 2003, 80.

Anonymous. 'Concepts of Health and Disease' *Journal of Medicine and Philosophy* 1, no. 3, special issue (1976).

Anonymous. 'Ex-star of Baywatch Has Contracted Hepatitis C.' *Globe and Mail*, 21 March 2002, A15.

Anonymous. 'Hepatitis C: Needles and Haystacks.' *The Economist*, 1 November 2003, 75–6.

Anonymous. 'The National Institutes of Health Consensus Development Conference: Management of Hepatitis C, Bethesda MD, 24 to 26 March 1997.' *Hepatology* 26, no. 3 Supplement 1 (1997): 1S–156S.

Anonymous. 'Reported Cases of Hepatitis A, B, and C in Canada – 1990–1999.' *Canada Communicable Disease Report* 20 supplement (2001): 24–5, 56–7, 110–11.

Aretaeus. *Extant Works of Aretaeus the Cappadocian*. Trans. F. Adams. London: Sydenham Society, 1856.

Arnaldus de Villanova. 'Tractatus de amore heroico [ca. 1280].' In *Arnaldi De Villanova Opera Medica Omnia*, vol. 3, ed. McVaugh, 1–54.

Aronowitz, Robert. *Making Sense of Illness: Science, Society, and Disease*. Cambridge: Cambridge University Press, 1998.

Asher, R., and D. Brissett. 'Codependency: A View from Women Married to Alcoholics.' *International Journal of Addictions* 23 (1988): 331–50.

Atkinson, Paul. *The Clinical Experience: The Construction and Reconstruction of Medical Reality*. Westmead, UK: Gower, 1981.

Austern, Linda Phyllis. '"For Love's a Good Musician": Performance, Audition, and Erotic Disorders in Early Modern Europe.' *Musical Quarterly* 82 (1998): 614–53.

– 'Musical Treatments for Lovesickness.' In *Music as Medicine: The History of Music Therapy since Antiquity*, ed. Peregrine Horden, 213–45. Aldershot: Ashgate, 2000.

Avicenna (Ibn Sina). 'De Ilisci. Insania ex amoribus.' *Liber Canonis de Medicinis*, Liber 3, Tract 4, cap 22. Brussels: Editions Culture et Civilisation, facsimile of Venice 1527 edition ed., 1971, 151v–152r.

Ayanian, John Z., and Arnold M. Epstein. 'Differences in the Use of

Procedures between Women and Men Hospitalized for Coronary Heart Disease.' *New England Journal of Medicine* 325 (1991): 221–5.

Baker, H.W. 'Needle Aspiration Biopsy (Hayes E. Martin).' *Ca: A Cancer Journal for Clinicians* 36 (1986): 69–70.

Bang, Nils, Paul Ruegsegger, Allyn B. Ley, and John S. LaDue. 'Detection of Hepatitis Carriers by Serum Glutamic Oxalacetic Transaminase.' *JAMA* 171 (1959): 2303–6.

Barker, Lewellys F., and Robert J. Gerety. 'The Clinical Problem of Hepatitis Transmission.' *Progress in Clinical and Biological Research* 11 (1976): 163–82.

Bartels, Andreas, and Semir Zeki. 'The Neural Basis of Romantic Love.' *Neuroreport* 11 (2000): 3829–34.

Baumann, E.D. 'Die pseudohippokratische Schrift "Peri Manies."' *Janus* 42 (1938): 129–41.

Bayer, Ronald. 'Politics, Science and the Problem of Psychiatric Nomenclature: A Case Study of the American Psychiatric Association Referendum on Homosexuality.' In *Scientific Controversies*, ed. Englehardt and Caplan, 381–400.

Beck, Ulrich, and Elisabeth Beck-Gernsheim, *The Normal Chaos of Love*. Cambridge: Polity Press, 1995.

Beecher, Donald. 'Erotic Love and the Inquisition: Jacques Ferrand and the Tribunal of Toulouse, 1620.' *Sixteenth Century Journal* 20 (1989): 41–53.

Beecher, Donald, and Massimo Ciavolella, eds. *Eros and Anteros: The Medical Traditions of Love in the Renaissance*. University of Toronto Italian Studies no. 9. Ottawa: Dovehouse Press, 1992.

Beeson, Paul B. 'Jaundice Occurring One to Four Months after Transfusion of Blood or Plasma: Report of Seven Cases.' *JAMA* 121 (1943): 1332–4.

Benady, Susannah. 'Alcohol a Major Predictor of Hepatitis C Recovery.' *Medical Post*, 15 May 2001, 7.

Benn, J. Miriam. *The Predicaments of Love*. London: Pluto Press, 1992.

Berman, Elaine S. '"Too Little Bone": The Medicalization of Osteoporosis.' *Journal of Women's Health and Law* 1, no. 3 (2000): 257–77.

Berrios, G.E. 'The Psychopathology of Affectivity: Conceptual and Historical Aspects.' *Psychological Medicine* 15 (1985): 745–58.

Bieber, Irving. 'On Arriving at the American Psychiatric Association

Decision on Homosexuality.' In *Scientific Controversies*, ed. Englehardt and Caplan, 417–36.

Biering, Páll. '"Codependency": A Disease or the Root of Nursing Excellence?' *Journal of Holistic Nursing* 16 (1998): 320–37.

Biernacka, Magdelena. 'History of Visceroptosis.' Unpublished paper read at the annual meeting of the Royal College of Physicians and Surgeons of Canada, Halifax, 1996.

Biesterfeldt, Hans-Hinrich, and Dimitri Gutas. 'The Malady of Love.' *Journal of the American Oriental Society* 104 (1984): 21–55.

Birchard, Karen. 'Study Confirms That Love Can Make You Crazy.' *Medical Post*, 6 April 1999, 63.

Blajchman, Morris. Interviews, 23 October 2002 and 20 December 2002.

Blajchman, M.A., S.B. Bull, and S.V. Feinman. 'Post Transfusion Hepatitis: Impact of Non-A, Non-B Surrogate Tests. Canadian Post-Transfusion Hepatitis Prevention Study.' *Lancet* 345 (1995): 21–5.

Blajchman, M.A., S.V. Feinman, and S.B. Bull. 'The Incidence of Post-Transfusion Hepatitis.' *New England Journal of Medicine* 328 (1993): 1280–1.

Blajchman, Morris A., and Harvey G. Klein. 'Looking Back in Anger.' *Transfusion Medicine Reviews* 11 (1997): 1–5.

Blanchette, Victor, Irwin Walker, Peter Gill, Margaret Adams, Robin Roberts, and Martin Inwood. 'Hepatitis C Infection in Patients with Hemophilia: Results of a National Survey. Canadian Hemophilia Clinic Directors Group.' *Transfusion Medicine Reviews* 8 (1994): 210–17.

Blumberg, Baruch S., Harvey J. Alter, and Sam Visnich. 'A "New" Antigen in Leukemia Sera.' *JAMA* 191 (1965): 541–6.

Blumberg, Baruch S., B.J. Gerstley, D.A. Hungerford, W. Thomas London, and Alton I. Sutnick. 'A Serum Antigen (Australia Antigen) in Down's Syndrome, Leukemia, and Hepatitis.' *Annals of Internal Medicine* 66 (1967): 924–31.

Blumberg, Baruch S., Irving Millman, and W. Thomas London. 'Ted Slavin's Blood and the Development of HBV Vaccine.' *New England Journal of Medicine* 312 (1985): 189.

Bonduelle, Michel, Toby Gelfand, and Christopher G. Goetz. *Charcot: Constructing Neurology*. New York: Oxford University Press, 1995.

Botté, C., and C. Janot. 'Epidemiology of HCV Infection in the General

Population and in Blood Transfusion.' *Nephrology Dialysis Transplantation* 11, Supplement 4 (1996): 19–21.

Bowden, D. Scott, Len D. Moaven, and Stephen A. Locarini. 'New Hepatitis Viruses: Are There Enough Letters in the Alphabet?' *Medical Journal of Australia* 164 (1996): 87–9.

Bradford, Dr. John. 'Pedophilia: Horrifying, But Is It a Crime?' *Globe and Mail*, 20 November 2000, A19.

Bradley, D.W. 'Studies of Non-A, Non-B Hepatitis and Characterization of the Hepatitis C Virus in Chimpanzees.' *Current Topics in Microbiology and Immunology* 242 (2000): 1–23.

Bradley, D.W., E.H. Cook, J.E. Maynard, K.A. McCaustland, J.W. Ebert, G.H. Dolana, R.A. Petzel, R.J. Kantor, A. Heilbrunn, H.A. Fields, and B.L. Murphy. 'Experimental Infection of Chimpanzees with Antihemophilic (Factor VIII) Materials: Recovery of Virus-Like Particles Associated with Non-A, Non-B hepatitis.' *Journal of Medical Virology* 3 (1979): 253–69.

Bradley, D.W., Krysztof Krawczynski, Michael J. Beach, and Michael A. Purdy. 'Non-A, Non-B Hepatitis. Toward the Discovery of Hepatitis C and E Viruses.' *Seminars in Liver Disease* 11 (1991): 128–46.

Bradley, D.W., J.E. Maynard, H. Popper, J.W. Ebert, E.H. Cook, H.A. Fields, and B.J. Kemler. 'Persistent Non-A, Non-B Hepatitis in Experimentally Infected Chimpanzees.' *Journal of Infectious Diseases* 143 (1981): 210–18.

Braverman, I., D. Wexler, and M. Oren. 'A Novel Mode of Infection with Hepatitis B: Penetrating Bone Fragments Due to the Explosion of a Suicide Bomber.' *Israel Medical Association Journal* 4 (2002): 528–9.

Bresters, D., E.P. Mauser-Bunschoten, H.W. Reesink, G. Roosendaal, C. L. van der Poel, R.A. Chamuleau, P.L.M. Jansen, C.J. Weegink, H.T.M. Cuypers, P.N. Lelie, and H.M. Van de Berg. 'Sexual Transmission of Hepatitis C Virus.' *Lancet* 342 (1993): 210–11.

Brock, Arthur John. *Greek Medicine, Being Extracts Illustrative of Medical Writers from Hippocrates to Galen*. London and Toronto: J.M. Dent and Sons, 1929.

Brooten, Bernadette. *Love between Women: Early Christian Responses to Female Homoeroticism*. Chicago and London: University of Chicago Press, 1996.

Brown, W. Miller. 'On Defining "Disease."' *Journal of Medicine and Philosophy* 10 (1985): 311–28.

Brumberg, Joan Jacobs, *Fasting Girls: The Emergence of Anorexia Nervosa as a Modern Disease*. Cambridge, MA: Harvard University Press, 1988.

Brundage, James A. *Sex, Law, and Marriage in the Middle Ages*. Aldershot, UK, and Brookfield, VT: Ashgate, 1993.

Bürgel, J.C. 'Love, Lust, and Longing: Eroticism in Early Islam as Reflected in Literary Sources.' In *Sixth Giorgio Levi della Vida Biennial Conference, Society and the Sexes in Medieval Islam*, ed. A.L. al-Sayyid-Marsot, 81–117. Malibu: Undena Press, 1979.

Bürgel, Johann Christoph 'Der Topos der Liebeskrankheit in der klassichen Dichtung des Islam.' In *Liebe als Krankheit*, ed. Stemmler, 75–104.

Burr, Chandler. *A Separate Creation: The Search for the Biological Origins of Sexual Orientation*. New York: Hyperion, 1996.

Buteau, Jacques, Allain D. Lesage, and Margaret C. Kiely. 'Homicide Followed by Suicide: A Quebec Case Series, 1988–1990.' *Canadian Journal of Psychiatry* 38 (1993): 552–6.

Butler, Declan. 'Verdict in French Blood Trial Shames Science.' *Nature* 359 (1992): 764.

Bynum, Bill. 'Discarded Diagnoses: Lovesickness.' *Lancet* 357 (2001): 403.

Bynum, William F. and Roy Porter, eds. *Medicine and the Five Senses*. Cambridge: Cambridge University Press, 1993.

Caelius Aurelianus. *De morbis acutis; De morbis chronicas. On Acute Diseases and On Chronic Diseases*. Trans. I.E. Drabkin. Chicago: University of Chicago Press, 1950.

Calabrese, Michael. 'The Lover's Cure in Ovid's *Remedia amoris* and Chaucer's *Miller's Tale*.' *English Language Notes* 32 (1994): 13–18.

Caldera de Heredia, Gaspard. *Tribunal medicum, magicum, et politicum. De prognosi fallacia in communi et particulari*. Lugduni Batavorum: Joannes Elsevierum, 1658.

Callum, Jeannie L., Peter H. Pinkerton, Ahmed S. Coovadia, Anne E. Thomson, and Frankie Dewsbury. 'An Evaluation of the Process and Costs Associated with Targeted Lookbacks for HCV and General Notification of Transfusion Recipients.' *Transfusion* 40 (2000): 1169–75.

Campbell, Fiona A.K. 'Inciting Legal Fictions: "Disability's" Date with Ontology and the Ableist Body of the Law.' *Griffith Law Review* 10 (2001): 42–62.

Canadian Legal Information Institute. *Attorney General of Canada v. Horace Krever* (1996–06–07) FC T-154–96. http://www.canlii.org/ca/cas/fct/1996/1996fct10032.html (accessed 11 February 2005).

Canadian Press Newswire. 'Red Cross Centre Sent out Possibly Deadly Blood While It Had Safe Blood.' 21 October 1994.

Canguilhem, Georges. *On the Normal and the Pathological*. Trans. Carolyn R. Fawcett and Robert S. Cohen. New York: Zone Books, 1989.

Caplan, Arthur L.H., Tristram Englehardt Jr, and James McCartney, eds. *Concepts of Health and Disease: Interdisciplinary Perspectives*. Reading, MA: Addison-Wesley, 1981.

Carotenuto, Aldo. *Eros and Pathos: Shades of Love and Suffering*. Trans. Charles Nopar. Toronto: Inner City Books, 1989.

Carson, Anne. *Eros the Bittersweet*. Princeton: Princeton University Press, 1986.

Carter, K. Codell. *The Rise of Causal Concepts of Disease: Case Histories*. Aldershot: Ashgate, 2003.

Cassell, Eric. 'Ideas in Conflict: The Rise and Fall (and Rise and Fall) of New Views of Disease.' *Daedalus* 115 (spring 1986): 19–41.

Celani, David. *The Illusion of Love: Why the Battered Woman Returns to Her Abuser*. New York: Columbia University Press, 1994.

Cellard, André. *Histoire de la folie au Québec de 1600 à 1850: le désordre*. Montreal: Boreal, 1991.

Celsus. *De Medicina, with an English Translation*. 3 vols. Trans. W.G. Spencer, 1: 272–3. London and Cambridge: Loeb Classical Library, Heinemann and Harvard University Press, 1960.

Cermak, Timmen L. 'Diagnostic Criteria for Codependency.' *Journal of Psychoactive Drugs* 18 (1986): 15–20.

Chastel, C. 'La peste de Barcelone. Epidémie de fièvre jaune de 1821.' *Bulletin de la Société de Pathologie Exotique* 92, no. 5, pt 2 (1999): 405–7.

Chauveau, P. 'Epidemiology of Hepatitis C Virus Infection in Chronic Hemodialysis.' *Nephrology, Dialysis, Transplantation* 11, Supplement 4 (1996): 39–41.

Chessick, Richard D. 'Malignant Eroticized Countertransference.' *Journal of the American Academy of Psychoanalysis* 25 (1997): 219–35.

Chiong, Miguel A. 'Dr. Carlos Finlay and Yellow Fever.' *CMAJ* 141 (1989): 1126.

Choo, Qui Lim, George Kuo, Amy J. Weiner, Lacy R. Overby, Daniel W. Bradley, and Michael Houghton. 'Isolation of a cDNA Clone Derived from a Blood-Borne Non-A Non-B Viral Hepatitis Genome.' *Science* 244 (1989): 359–61.

Ciavolella, Massimo. *La malattia d'amore dall'antichità al medioevo.* Rome: Bulzoni, 1976.

– 'Mediaeval Medicine and Arcite's Love Sickness.' *Florilegium* 1 (1979): 222–41.

Cicero, Marcus Tullius. 'Tusculan Disputationes, IV.' In *Tusculan Disputationes. Loeb Classical Library.* Trans. J.E. King. Cambridge, MA, and London: Harvard University Press and Heinemann, 1971.

Comfort, Alex, ed., *The Joy of Sex: A Cordon Bleu Guide to Lovemaking.* New York: Simon and Schuster, 1972.

– *The Joy of Sex: A Gourmet Guide to Lovemaking.* New York: Crown Publishers, 1972.

Connor, Joan. 'How to Stop Loving Someone: A Twelve-Step Program.' *TriQuarterly* 98 (winter 1996–7): 167–76.

Constantine the African. 'Viaticum I.20 [ca. 1180–1200].' In *Lovesickness in the Middle Ages,* ed. Wack, 179–93.

Cook, Donna Lynn, and Kimberly R. Barber. 'Relationship between Social-Support, Self-Esteem, and Codependency in the African American Female.' *Journal of Cultural Diversity* 4 (1997): 32–8.

Cooke, Robert E. 'Vulnerable Children.' In *Children as Research Subjects: Science, Ethics, and Law,* ed. Michael A. Grodin and Leonard H. Glantz, 193–214. New York and Oxford: Oxford University Press, 1994.

Corvisart des Marets, Jean-Nicolas. *An Essay on the Organic Diseases and Lesions of the Heart and Great Vessels.* Trans. Jacob Gates. New York: Hafner Publishing House, [1806] 1962.

Couroucé, Anne-Marie. 'De l'hépatite Non-A Non-B à l'hépatite C.' *Transfusion Clinique et Biologique* 4 (1997): 287–90.

Cousins, Norman. 'The Anatomy of an Illness (as Perceived by the Patient).' *New England Journal of Medicine* 295 (1976): 1458–63.

Crozier, Ivan. '"Rough Winds Do Shake the Darling Buds of May": William Acton and the Sexuality of the Child.' Unpublished paper read at 'Health and the Child; Care and Culture in History,' Geneva, 13–15 September 2001.

Cullen, William. *Apparatus ad nosologiam methodicam seu Synopsis nosologiae methodicae in usu studiosorum.* Amstelodami: Fratrum de Tournes, 1775.

Cyrino, Monica Silveira. *In Pandora's Jar: Lovesickness in Early Greek Poetry.* Lanham, MD: University Press of America, 1995.

Davis, Audrey B. *Medicine and Its Technology. An Introduction to the History of Medical Instrumentation.* Westport, CT, and London: Greenwood, 1981.

Delaporte, François. *The History of Yellow Fever: An Essay on the Birth of Tropical Medicine.* Cambridge, MA, and London: MIT Press, 1991.

Desforges, Jane F. 'AIDS and Preventive Treatment in Hemophilia.' *New England Journal of Medicine* 308 (1983): 94–5.

De Vos, R., C. Verslype, E. Depla, J. Fevery, B. Van Damme, V. Desmet, and T. Roskams. Ultrastructural Visualization of Hepatitis C Virus Components in Human and Primate Liver Biopsies.' *Journal of Hepatology* 37 (2002): 370–9.

Diagnostic and Statistical Manual of Mental Disorders: DSM–IIIR. 3rd rev. ed. Washington, DC: American Psychiatric Association, 1987.

Diagnostic and Statistical Manual of Mental Disorders: DSM–IV. 4th ed. Washington, DC: American Psychiatric Association, 1994.

Dietzman, Dale E., James Harnisch, C. George Ray, E. Russell Alexander, and King K. Holmes. 'Hepatitis B Surface Antigen (HBsAg) and Antibody to HBsAg. Prevalence in Homosexual and Heterosexual Men.' *JAMA* 238 (1977): 2625–6.

Dijkstra, Bram. *Idols of Perversity: Fantasies of Feminine Evil in Fin-de-Siècle Culture.* New York and Oxford: Oxford University Press, 1986.

Dritz, Selma K. 'Medical Aspects of Homosexuality.' *New England Journal of Medicine* 302 (1980): 463–4.

Dronke, Peter. *Medieval Latin and the Rise of the European Love-Lyric* (Oxford: Clarendon, 1968).

Drossman, Douglas A., Jane Leserman, Ginette Nachman, Zhiming Li, Honi Gluck, Timothy C. Tommey, and C. Madeline Mitchell. 'Sexual and Physical Abuse in Women with Functional or Organic Gastrointestinal Disorders.' *Annals of Internal Medicine* 113 (1990): 828–33.

Drossman, Douglas A., Nicholas J Talley, Jane Leserman, Kevin W.

Olden, and Marcelo A. Barreiro. 'Sexual and Physical Abuse in Gastrointestinal Illness; Review and Recommendations.' *Annals of Internal Medicine* 123 (1995): 782–94.

Du Laurens, André. *Les oeuvres de M. André Du Laurens*, 2 parts in one volume. Paris: Nicolas et Jean Lacoste, 1646.

Duffin, Jacalyn. 'Grand Rounds; Osteodensosis.' *CMAJ* 165 (2001): 1609–11.

– 'The Great Canadian Peritonitis Debate, 1844–47.' *Histoire sociale / Social History* 19 (1987): 407–24.

– 'Sick Doctors: Bayle and Laennec on Their Own Phthisis.' *Journal of the History of Medicine* 43 (1988): 165–82.

– 'Why Does Cirrhosis Belong to Laennec?' *CMAJ* 137 (1987): 393–6.

Duminil, Marie-Paule. 'La mélancholie amoureuse dans l'antiquité.' In *La folie et le corps*, ed. J. Céard, 91–110. Paris: Presses de l'École Normale Supérieure, 1985.

Engel, George L. 'The Need for a New Medical Model: A Challenge for Biomedicine.' In *Concepts of Health and Disease*, ed. Caplan et al., 589–607.

– 'A Unified Concept of Health and Disease.' *Perspectives in Biology and Medicine* 3 (1960): 459–85.

Englehardt, H.T. 'The Disease of Masturbation: Values and the Concept of Disease.' *Bulletin of the History of Medicine* 48 (1974): 234–48.

Englehardt, H. Tristram, and Arthur L. Caplan, eds. *Scientific Controversies: Case Studies in the Resolution and Closure of Disputes in Science and Technology.* Cambridge: Cambridge University Press, 1987.

Enouch, M. David, and W.H. Trethown. *Uncommon Psychiatric Syndromes.* Bristol: John Wright and Sons, 1979.

Epstein, J.B., G. Rea, C.H. Sherlock, and R.G. Mathias. 'Continuing Investigation and Controversy Regarding Risk of Transmission of Infection via Dental Handpieces.' *Journal of the Canadian Dental Association / Journal de l'Association Dentaire Canadienne* 62 (1996): 485–91.

Ergun, Gulchin A., and Paul F. Miskovitz. 'Viral Hepatitis. The New ABC's.' *Postgraduate Medicine* 88 (1990): 69–76.

Esquirol, J.E.D. *Mental Maladies. A Treatise on Insanity.* Trans. E.K. Hunt. New York and London: Hafner, [1845] 1965.

Eyster, M. Elaine, Harvey J. Alter, Louis M. Aledort, Stella Quan, Angelos Hatzakis, and James J. Goedert. 'Heterosexual Co-Transmission of Hepatitis C Virus (HCV) and Human Immunodeficiency Virus (HIV).' *Annals of Internal Medicine* 115 (1991): 764–8.

Farley, John. *Bilharzia: A History of Imperial Tropical Medicine.* Cambridge: Cambridge University Press, 1991.

Farmer, Sally A. 'Entitlement in Codependency: Developmental and Therapeutic Considerations.' *Journal of Addictive Diseases* 18 (1999): 55–68.

Faulkner, R.O., Edward F. Wente, and William Kelly Simpson, eds. *The Literature of Ancient Egypt.* New Haven, CT, and London: Yale University Press, 1973.

Feinman, S.V., B. Berris, and S. Bojarski. 'Postransfusion Hepatitis in Toronto, Canada.' *Gastroenterology* 95 (1988): 464–9.

Feinstone, Stephen M,. Albert Z. Kapikan, and Robert H. Purcell. 'Hepatitis A: Detection by Immune Electron Microscopy of a Viruslike Antigen Associated with Acute Illness.' *Science* 182 (1973): 1026–8.

Feinstone, Stephen M., Albert Z. Kapikan, Robert H. Purcell, Harvey J. Alter, and Paul V. Holland. 'Transfusion-Associated Hepatitis Not Due to Viral Hepatitis Type A or B.' *New England Journal of Medicine* 292 (1975): 767–70.

Feldberg, Georgina. *Disease and Class: Tuberculosis and the Shaping of Modern North American Society.* New Brunswick, NJ: Rutgers University Press, 1995.

Fernández, Julia Blanco. 'El amor hereos en La Celestina: la prescripción de Celestina.' MA thesis, McGill University, 1999.

Ferrand, Jacques. *A Treatise on Lovesickness.* Trans. and ed. Donald A. Beecher and Massimo Ciavolella. Syracuse: Syracuse University Press, 1990.

Figlio, Karl. 'Chlorosis and Chronic Disease in Nineteenth-Century Britain: The Social Constitution of Somatic Illness in a Capitalist Society.' *Social History* 3 (1978): 167–97.

Fleck, Ludwik. *Genesis and Development of a Scientific Fact.* Chicago: University of Chicago Press, 1979.

Fluker, J.L. 'A 10-Year Study of Homosexually Transmitted Infection.' *British Journal of Venereal Diseases* 52 (1976): 155–60.

Fontaine, Marie-Madeleine. 'La lignée des commentaires à la chanson de Guido Cavalcanti "Donna me prega": évolution des relations entre philosophie, médecine, et littérature dans le débat sur la nature d'amour (de la fin de XIIIe siècle à celle du XVIe).' In *La folie et le corps*, ed. J. Céard, 159–78. Paris: Presses de l'École Normale Supérieure, 1985.

Ford, P.M., C. White, H. Kaufmann, J. MacTavish, M. Pearson, S. Ford, P.S. Mistry, and P. Connop. 'Voluntary Anonymous Linked Study of the Prevalence of HIV Infection and Hepatitis C among Inmates in a Canadian Federal Penitentiary for Women.' *CMAJ* 153 (1995): 1605–9.

– 'Voluntary Screening for Hepatitis C in a Canadian Federal Penitentiary for Men.' *Canada Communicable Disease Report* 21 (1995): 134–5.

Fortenbaugh, W.W. *Aristotle on Emotions*. London: Duckworth, 1975.

Foucault, Michel. *Naissance de la clinique: une archéologie du regard médical*. Paris: Presses Universitaires de France, 1963.

Frable, William J. 'Fine-Needle Aspiration Biopsy: A Review.' *Human Pathology* 14 (1983): 9–28.

Fracastoro, Girolamo. *Syphilis, or the French Disease*. Trans. Heneage Wynne-Finch. London: Heinemann, 1935.

Frösner, Gert G., Holger M. Buchholz, and Hans Joachim Gerth. 'Prevalence of Hepatitis B Antibody in Prostitutes.' *American Journal of Epidemiology* 102 (1975): 241–50.

Funke, Hermann. 'Greische und römische Antike.' In *Liebe als Krankheit*, ed. Stemmler, 11–30.

Galen. *De locis affectis. On the Affected Parts*. Trans. Rudolph E. Siegel. Basel and New York: Karger, 1976.

– *De propriorum animi cujusque affectuum dignotione et curatione. On the Passions and Errors of the Soul*. Trans. Paul W. Harkins. Columbus: Ohio State University Press, 1963.

– *Galeni de praecognitionae. Galen On Prognosis. Edition, Translation, and Commentary*. Ed. Vivian Nutton. Berlin: Corpus Medicorum Grecorum V 8, 1; Akademie Verlag, 1979.

– 'Galeni de praenotione ad Posthumum liber.' In *Opera Omnia*, vol. 14, ed. C.G. Kuhn, 630–5. Hildesheim: Georg Olms, 1965.

Garcia-Kutzbach, A. 'Medicine among the Ancient Maya.' *Southern Medical Journal* 69 (1976): 938–40.

Gaubius, Hieronymus David. *Institutiones pathologiae medicinalis*. Lipsiae: Joannis Pauli Krausii Bibliopolae Viennensis, 1759.

Gentilcore, David. 'Ritualized Illness and Music Therapy: Views of Tarantism in the Kingdom of Naples.' In *Music as Medicine: The His-*

tory of Music Therapy since Antiquity, ed. Peregrine Horden, 256–72. Aldershot: Ashgate, 2000.

Geppert, Alexander C.T. 'Divine Sex, Happy Marriage, Regenerated Nation: Marie Stopes's Marital Manual *Married Love* and the Making of a Best-Seller.' *Journal of the History of Sexuality* 8 (1998): 389–433.

Gherardini, M. R. 'Über Eine Gelbsuchtepidemie Während des Sommers 538 im Gebiet und Ancona.' *Gesnerus* 26 (1969): 145–53.

Giedke, Adelheid. 'Die Liebeskrankheit in der Geschichte der Medizin.' Dissertation zur Erlangung des Grades eines Doktors der Medizin. Universität Düsseldorf aus dem Institut für Geschichte der Medizin, 1983.

Gilman, Sander L. *Difference and Pathology: Stereotypes of Sexuality, Race, and Madness*. Ithaca, NY: Cornell University Press, 1985.

Ginzburg, Carlo. 'Clues: Roots of an Evidential Paradigm [1986].' In *Clues, Myths and the Historical Method*. Trans. John and Anne Tedeschi. Baltimore and London: Johns Hopkins University Press, 1989.

Giulivi, A., M.T. Aye, E. Gray, V. Scalia, P. Gill, and G. Cheng. 'Anti-Hepatitis C Virus (HCV) Screening at a Canadian Red Cross Center: Significance of a Positive c100 HCV Enzyme-Linked Immunosorbent Assay.' *Transfusion* 32 (1992): 309–11.

Goedert, J.J., M.G. Sarngadharan, M.E. Eyster, S.H. Weiss, A.J. Bodner, R.C. Gallo, and W.A. Blattner. 'Antibodies Reactive with Human T Cell Leukemia Viruses in the Serum of Hemophiliacs Receiving Factor VIII Concentrate.' *Blood* 65 (1985): 492–5.

Goldberg, Jeff. *Anatomy of a Scientific Discovery.* Toronto and New York: Bantam, 1988.

Goldman, Mindy, and Anne Long. 'Hepatitis C Lookback in Canada.' *Vox Sanguinis* 78 Supplement 2 (2000): 249–52.

Goldman, Mindy, and Gwendoline Spurll. 'Hepatitis C Lookback.' *Current Opinion in Hematology* 7 (2000): 392–6.

Gordon, Stuart C., Ashe H. Patel, Gregory W. Kulkesza, Robert Barnes, and Ann L. Silverman. 'Lack of Evidence for the Heterosexual Transmission of Hepatitis C.' *American Journal of Gastroenterology* 87 (1992): 1849–51.

Gotham, H.J., and K.J. Sher. 'Do Codependent Traits Involve More than Basic Dimensions of Personality and Psychopathology?' *Journal of Studies on Alcohol* 57 (1996): 34–9.

Gourevitch, Danielle. *Le triangle hippocratique dans le monde gréco-romain: le malade, sa maladie et son médecin.* Rome: École Française de Rome, 1984.

Gournay, Jérôme, Patrick Marcellin, Michèle Martinot-Peignoux, Claude Degott, Franck Gabriel, Françoise Courtois, Michel Branger, Anne Marie Wild, Serge Erlinger, and Jean-Pierre Benhamou. 'Hepatitis C Genotypes in French Blood Donors.' *Journal of Medical Virology* 45 (1995): 399–404.

Grant, Mark. *Dieting for an Emperor. A Translation of Books 1 and 4 of Oribasius' Medical Compilations with an Introduction and Commentary. Studies in Ancient Medicine,* vol. 15. Ed. John Scarborough. Leiden, New York, Köln: Brill, 1997.

Greenberg, Daniel. 'Out Goes the Surgeon General.' *Lancet* 344 (1994): 1760.

Grimbert, Joan Tasker. *'Voleir* vs. *Poeir*: Frustrated Desire in Thomas's *Tristan.'* *Philological Quarterly* 69 (1990): 153–65.

Grmek, Mirko D. 'Le concept de maladie.' In *Histoire de la pensée médicale en Occident.* Ed. Mirko D. Grmek and Bernardino Fantini. Vol. 1: *Antiquité et moyen âge* (Paris: Seuil, 1995), 211–26, and vol 2: *De la Renaissance aux Lumières* (Paris: Seuil, 1997), 157–76.

– 'Le concept de maladie émergente.' *History and Philosophy of the Life Sciences* 15 (1993): 281–96.

– *History of AIDS: Emergence and Origin of a Modern Pandemic.* Trans. Russell C. Maulitz and Jacalyn Duffin. Princeton: Princeton University Press, 1990.

– *Les maladies à l'aube de la civilisation occidentale.* Paris: Payot, 1983.

– *La vie, les maladies, et l'histoire.* Ed. Louise L. Lambrichs. Paris: Seuil, 2001.

Grossman, Dave, and Gloria Degaetano. *Stop Teaching Our Kids to Kill.* New York: Crown Publishers, 1999.

Guardiani, Francesco. 'Eros and Misogyny from Giovan Battista Marino to Ferrante Pallavicino.' In *Eros and Anteros*, ed. Beecher and Ciavolella, 147–59.

Gugler, MaryBeth. 'Mercury and the "Pains of Love" in Jonathan Swift's "A Beautiful Young Nymph Going to Bed."' *English Language Notes* 20 (1991): 31–6.

Guild, Rob. 'Hep C Victim Fights for Compensation: Man Denied Money over Adolescent Indiscretion with Intravenous Drug.' *Toronto Star*, 13 December 1999, A6.

Gunby, P. 'Clinical Trial of Vaccine for Type B Hepatitis to Begin Next Month.' *JAMA* 241 (1979): 979–80.

Haage, Bernhard D. '"Amor hereos" als medizinischer terminus technicus in der Antike und im Mittelalter.' In *Liebe als Krankheit*, ed. Stemmler, 31–74.

Hacking, Ian. *Rewriting the Soul: Multiple Personality and the Sciences of Memory*. Princeton, NJ: Princeton University Press, 1995.

Haddad, Tony, ed. *Men and Masculinities: A Critical Anthology*. Toronto: Canadian Scholars' Press, 1993.

Hamann, Stephan B., Timothy D. Ely, Scott T. Grafton, and Clinton D. Kilts. 'Amygdala Activity Related to Enhanced Memory for Pleasant and Aversive Stimuli.' *Nature Neuroscience* 2 (1999): 289–93.

Hamer, Dean H. 'Sexual Orientation [letter].' *Nature Neuroscience* 365 (1993): 702.

Hamer, Dean H., S. Hu, V.L. Magnuson, N. Hu, and A.M. Pattatucci. 'A Linkage between DNA Markers on the X Chromosome and Male Sexual Orientation.' *Science* 261 (1993): 321–7.

Hansen, Bert. 'American Physicians' "Discovery" of Homosexuals, 1880–1900: A New Diagnosis in a Changing Society.' In *Framing Disease*, ed. Rosenberg and Golden, 104–33.

Harley, David. 'Rhetoric and the Social Construction of Sickness and Healing.' *Social History of Medicine* 12 (1999): 407–35.

Harlow, John. 'Limits of Love: A Many Splendored 2 1/2 years.' *Montreal Gazette*, 25 July 1999, A1, A6.

– 'Love Is about 30 Months, Tops.' *Toronto Star*, 25 July 1999, A1.

Harper, Jeane, and Connie Capdevila. 'Codependency: A Critique.' *Journal of Psychoactive Drugs* 22 (1990): 285–92.

Hatfield, E., and S. Sprecher. 'Measuring Passionate Love in Intimate Relationships.' *Journal of Adolescence* 9, no. 4 (1986): 383–410.

Heddle, Nancy, John G. Kelton, Fiona Smaill, Krista Foss, Jennifer Everson, Cynthia Janzen, Chris Walker, Marak Jones, and Debby Hammons. 'A Canadian Hospital-Based HIV/Hepatitis Look-Back Notification Program.' *CMAJ* 157 (1997): 149–54.

Hefferman, Carol Falvo. *The Melancholy Muse: Chaucer, Shakespeare, and Early Medicine.* Pittsburgh: Duquesnne University Press, 1995.

Hesiod. 'Theogony.' In *Hesiod.* Trans. Richmond Lattimore. Ann Arbor: University of Michigan Press, 1959.

Hill, Joanna M., William L. Farrar, and Candace B. Pert. 'Autoradiographic Localization of T4 Antigen, the HIV Receptor, in Human Brain.' *International Journal of Neuroscience* 32 (1987): 687–93.

Hippocrate. *Oeuvres complètes d'Hippocrate.* 10 vols. Trans. Emile Littré. Paris: Baillière, 1839–1861.

Hippocrates. *Hippocrates with an English Translation. Loeb Classical Library.* 8 vols. Trans. W.H.S. Jones, E. Withington, Paul Potter, and Wesley D. Smith. London: Heinemann; Cambridge, MA: Harvard University Press, 1923–95.

– 'The Sacred Disease.' Trans. John Chadwick and W.H. Mann. In *History of Medicine: Selected Readings.* Ed. Lester S. King, 54–61. Harmondsworth: Penguin, 1971.

Hite, Shere. *The Hite Report: A Nationwide Study on Female Sexuality.* New York: Macmillan, 1976.

– *The Hite Report on Male Sexuality.* New York: Knopf, 1981.

Hoffman, Werner. 'Liebe als Krankheit in der mittelhochdeutschen Lyrik.' In *Liebe als Krankheit*, ed. Stemmler, 221–57.

Hollander, Robert. *Boccaccio's Two Venuses.* New York: Columbia University Press, 1977.

Holmes, Gary (and 15 other authors). 'Chronic Fatigue Syndrome: A Working Case Definition.' *Annals of Internal Medicine* 108 (1988): 387–9.

Homer. *The Odyssey of Homer.* Trans. and ed. Richmond Lattimore. New York: Harper Row, 1965, 1967.

Hoofnagle, J.H., R.J. Gerety, J. Thiel, and L.F. Barker. 'The Prevalence of Hepatitis B Surface Antigen in Commercially Prepared Plasma Products.' *Journal of Laboratory and Clinical Medicine* 88 (1976): 102–13.

Hoofnagle, Jay H., Robert J. Gerety, Edward Tabor, Stephen M. Feinstone, Lewellys F. Barker, and Robert H. Purcell. 'Transmission of Non-A, Non-B Hepatitis.' *Annals of Internal Medicine* 87 (1977): 14–20.

Horrigan, Bonnie. 'Candace Pert, Ph.D.: Neuropeptides, AIDS, and the Science of Mind-Body Healing.' *Alternative Therapies in Health and Medicine* 1 (1995): 70–6.

Howard, Lloyd. 'Dino's Interpretation of "Donna me prega" and Cavalcanti's "Canzoniere."' *Canadian Journal of Italian Studies* 6 (1983): 167–82.

Howell, Joel D. *Technology in the Hospital: Transforming Patient Care in the Early Twentieth Century.* Baltimore: Johns Hopkins University, 1995.

Hudson, Robert. 'The Biography of Disease: Lessons from Chlorosis.' *Bulletin of the History of Medicine* 51 (1977): 448–63.

– *Disease and Its Control; the Shaping of Modern Thought.* Westport, CT: Greenwood, 1980.

Hughes-Hammer, Cyrilla, Donna S. Martsolf, and Richard A. Zeller. 'Depression and Codependency in Women.' *Archives of Psychiatric Nursing* 12 (1998): 326–34.

Humphreys, Margaret. *Yellow Fever and the South.* New Brunswick, NJ: Rutgers University Press, 1992.

Hurcom, Carolyn, Alex Copello, and Jim Orford. 'The Family and Alcohol; Effects of Excessive Drinking and Conceptualizations of Spouses over Recent Decades.' *Substance Use and Misuse* 35 (2000): 473–502.

Irwin, H.J. 'Codependence, Narcissism, and Childhood Trauma.' *Journal of Clinical Psychology* 51 (1995): 658–65.

Jackson, Stanley W. *Melancholia and Depression: From Hippocratic Times to Modern Times.* New Haven, CT: Yale University Press, 1986.

Jacquart, Danielle. 'L'amour "héroique" à travers le traité d'Arnaud de Villeneuve.' In *La folie et le corps,* ed. J. Céard, 143–58. Paris: Presses de l'École Normale Supérieure, 1985.

Jacquart, Danielle, and Claude Thomasset. *Sexuality and Medicine in the Middle Ages.* Trans. Matthew Adamson. Princeton: Princeton University Press, 1988.

Johnson, Hillary. *Osler's Web: Inside the Labyrinth of the Chronic Fatigue Syndrome.* New York: Penguin, 1996.

Jones, S.L. 'Are We Addicted to Codependency?' *Archives of Psychiatric Nursing* 5 (1991): 55–6.

Josephson, Wendy L. *Television Violence: A Review of the Effects on Children of Different Ages.* Ottawa: Department of Canadian Heritage and Health Canada, 1995.

Kaiser, Jocelyn. 'No Misconduct in "Gay Gene" Study.' *Science* 275 (1997): 1251.

Karnein, Alfred. '*Amor est passio*: A Definition of Courtly Love.' In *Court and Poet: Selected Proceedings of the Third Congress of the International Courtly Literature Society*, ed. Glynn S. Burgess, 215–21. Liverpool: Francis Cairns, 1981.

Keele, Kenneth D. *The Evolution of Clinical Methods in Medicine*. Springfield, IL: Charles C. Thomas, 1963.

Kerr, Grant. 'Roy Arrested after Domestic Row.' *Globe and Mail*, 23 October 2000, A1, A14.

Kevles, Bettyann. *Naked to the Bone: Medical Imaging in the Twentieth Century*. New Brunswick, NJ: Rutgers University Press, 1997.

Khairallah, A.E. *Love, Madness, and Poetry. An Interpretation of the Magnun Legend*. Beirut: Beiruter Texte und Studien, Band 25, 1980.

Kim, Evelyn. 'A Brief History of Chronic Fatigue Syndrome.' *JAMA* 272 (1994): 1070–1.

King, Helen. '"Green Sickness": Hippocrates, Galen, and the Origins of the Disease of Virgins.' *International Journal of the Classical Tradition* 2 (1996): 372–87.

King, Lester S. 'Boissier de Sauvages and 18th-Century Nosology.' *Bulletin of the History of Medicine* 40 (1966): 43–51.

– *Medical Thinking: A Historical Preface*. Princeton, NJ: Princeton University Press, 1982.

– *The Medical World of the Eighteenth Century*. Chicago: University of Chicago Press, 1958.

– *The Road to Medical Enlightenment*. London and New York: Macdonald and American Elsevier, 1970.

Kinsey, Alfred C. *Sexual Behavior in the Human Male*. Philadephia: Saunders, 1948.

– *Sexual Behavior in the Human Female*. Philadelphia: Saunders, 1953.

Klibansky, Raymond, Erwin Panofsky, and Fritz Saxl. *Saturn and Melancholy: Studies in the History of Natural Philosophy, Religion, and Art*. Cambridge and London: Nelson, 1964.

Kondro, Wayne. 'Canada's Hepatitis C Compensation Derailed.' *Lancet* 351 (1998): 1415.

– 'Compensation for Canada's Hepatitis C Victims to Be Re-Evaluated.' *Lancet* 351 (1998): 1567.

– 'Curtailed Canadian HIV Compensation.' *Lancet* 343 (1994): 783–4.

– 'Revelations Rock Canada's Tainted-Blood Inquiry.' *Lancet* 347 (1996): 1178.
– 'Revised Estimates of Hepatitis C from Tainted Blood Published.' *Lancet* 352 (1998): 466.
Koziol, D.E., P.V. Holland, D.W. Alling, J.C. Melpolder, R.E. Solomon, R.H. Purcell, L.M. Hudson, F.J. Shoup, H. Krakauer, and H.J. Alter. 'Antibody to Hepatitis B Core Antigen as a Paradoxical Marker for Non-A, Non-B Hepatitis Agents in Donated Blood.' *Annals of Internal Medicine* 104 (1986): 488–95.
Kramer, Peter D. *Listening to Prozac: A Psychiatrist Explores Antidepressant Drugs and the Remaking of Self.* New York: Penguin, 1993.
Krever, Horace. *Commission of Inquiry on the Blood System in Canada. Final Report.* 3 vols. Ottawa: Canadian Government Publishing – PWGSC, 1997.
Krugman, Saul. 'The Willowbrook Hepatitis Studies Revisited: Ethical Aspects.' *Reviews of Infectious Diseases* 8 (1986): 157–62.
Krugman, Saul, Joan Giles, and Jack Hammond. 'Infectious Hepatitis. Evidence for Two Distinctive Clinical, Epidemiological, and Immunological Types of Infection.' *JAMA* 200 (1967): 365–73.
Kunitz, Stephen J. *Disease and Social Diversity: The European Impact on the Health of Non-Europeans.* New York: Oxford University Press, 1994.
Kuo, G., Q.L. Choo, H.J. Alter, G.L. Gitnick, A.G. Redeker, R.H. Purcell, T. Miyamura, J.L. Dienstag, M.J. Alter, C.E. Stevens. 'An Assay for Circulating Antibodies to a Major Etiologic Virus of Human Non-A, Non-B Hepatitis.' *Science* 244 (1989): 362–4.
Ladurie, Emannuel Le Roy. *Montaillou, village occitan de 1294 à 1324.* Paris: Gallimard, 1975.
Laennec, R.T.H. Leçons au Collège de France, 1822–23, Leçon 36, Musée Laennec, Nantes France, MS. Cl. 2 a(A), f. 14r–v.
Lamont, L.T. 'Postoperative Jaundice.' *Surgical Clinics of North America* 54 (1974): 637–45.
Lane, Richard D., Eric M. Reiman, Geoffrey L. Ahern, Gary E. Schwartz, and Richard J. Davidson. 'Neuroanatomical Correlates of Happiness, Sadness, and Disgust.' *American Journal of Psychiatry* 154 (1997): 926–33.
Langley, J.M., S.G. Squires, D.M. MacDonald, D. Anderson, K. Peltekian, and J.W. Scott. 'Evaluation of the Notification of Hepatitis

C Risk to Children Who Received Unscreened Blood or Blood Products.' *Communicable Disease and Public Health* 4 (2001): 288–92.

Laudenslager, Mark L., Susan M. Ryan, Richard Hyson, and Steven F. Maier. 'Coping and Immunosuppression: Inescapable but Not Escapable Shock Suppresses Lymphocyte Proliferation.' *Science* 221 (1983): 568–70.

Leavitt, Judith Walzer. *Brought to Bed: Childbearing in America, 1750 to 1950.* New York: Oxford University Press, 1986.

Leckman, James F. and Linda C. Mayes. 'Preoccupations and Behaviours Associated with Romantic and Parental Love.' *Child and Adolescent Psychiatric Clinics of North America* 8 (1999): 635–65.

Lederer, Susan, and Michael A. Grodin. 'Historical Overview: Pediatric Experimentation.' In *Children as Research Subjects: Science, Ethics, and Law,* ed. Michael A. Grodin and Leonard H. Glantz, 3–25. New York and Oxford: Oxford University Press, 1994.

Lefkowitz, Mary R., and Maureen B. Fant. *Women's Life in Greece and Rome: A Source Book in Translation.* 2nd ed. London: Duckworth, 1992.

Léger, Pierre. *La canadienne française et l'amour, ou l'homme démystifié.* Montreal: Éditions du Jour, 1965.

Lerner, Vladimir, Alexander Kapstan, and Eliezer Witztum. 'The Misidentification of Clerambault's and Kandinsky-Clerambault's Syndromes.' *Canadian Journal of Psychiatry* 46 (2001): 441–3.

Levene, Cyril, and Baruch S. Blumberg. 'Additional Specificities of Australia Antigen and the Possible Identification of Hepatitis Carriers.' *Nature* 221 (1969): 195–6.

Levor, M. 'Die Liebeskrankheit in Goethes Dichtung.' *Deutsche Medizinische Wochenschrift* 37 (1911): 220–2.

Lewis, C.S. *The Allegory of Love. A Study in Medieval Tradition.* Oxford and New York: Oxford University Press, 1936, 1990.

Lewis, M.E., M. Mishkin, E. Bragin, R.M. Brown, C.B. Pert, and A. Pert. 'Opiate Receptor Gradients in Monkey Cerebral Cortex: Correspondence with Sensory Processing Hierarchies.' *Science* 211 (1981): 1166–9.

Liang, T. Jake, Barbara Rehermann, Leonard B. Seeff, and Jay H. Hoofnagle. 'Pathogenesis, Natural History, Treatment, and Prevention of Hepatitis C.' *Annals of Internal Medicine* 132 (2000): 296–305.

Lindley, Natasha R., Peter J Giordano, and Elliott D. Hammer. 'Codependency: Predictors and Psychometric Issues.' *Journal of Clinical Psychology* 55 (1999): 59–64.

Long, A., G. Spurll, H. Demers, and M. Goldman. 'Targeted Hepatitis C Lookback: Quebec, Canada.' *Transfusion* 39 (1999): 194–200.

Loudon, Irvine S. 'Chlorosis, Anaemia, and Anorexia Nervosa.' *British Medical Journal* 281 (1980): 1669–75.

– 'The Disease Called Chlorosis.' *Psychological Medicine* 14 (1984): 27–36.

Lowes, John Livingston. 'The Loveres Maladye of Hereos.' *Modern Philology* 11 (1913–14): 491–546.

Lucian. *The Syrian Goddess (De dea Syria)*. Missoula, MT: Scholars Press for the Society of Biblical Literature, 1976.

Lukits, Ann. 'The Growing Numbers of Flat-Headed Babies.' *Kingston Whig-Standard*, 10 August 2002, 1, 11.

Lunman, Kim. 'Liver Transplant Hopes Rest on Prayer.' *Globe and Mail*, 4 November 2000, A4.

MacDonald, Jake. 'Doctor of Love.' *National Post*, 2 March 2002, SP1, SP6.

Maclean, Ian. *Logic, Signs and Nature in the Renaissance: The Case of Learned Medicine*. Cambridge: Cambridge University Press, 2002.

Malleson, Andrew. *Whiplash and Other Useful Illnesses*. Montreal and Kingston: McGill-Queen's University Press, 2002.

Malloy, Gail B., and Ann C. Berkery. 'Codependency: A Feminist Perspective.' *Journal of Psychosocial Nursing and Mental Health Services* 31 (1993): 15–19.

Marazziti, D., H.S. Akiskal, A. Rossi, and G.B. Cassano. 'Alteration of the Platelet Serotonin Transporter in Romantic Love.' *Psychological Medicine* 29 (1999): 741–5.

Marshall, Eliot. 'NIH's "Gay Gene" Study Questioned.' *Science* 268 (1995): 1841.

Martin, Julian. 'Sauvages's Nosology: Medical Enlightenment in Montpellier.' In *The Medical Enlightenment of the Eighteenth Century*, ed. Andrew Cunningham and Roger K. French, 111–37. Cambridge: Cambridge University Press, 1990.

Marzuk, Peter M., Kenneth Tardiff, and Charles S. Hirsch. 'The Epidemiology of Murder-Suicide.' *JAMA* 267 (1992): 3179–83.

Masters William H., and Virginia E. Johnson. *Human Sexual Response*. Boston: Little, Brown, 1966.

McArthur, Sean, and Marrie McKenna. '"Love Bug" Hits World's E-Mail.' *Globe and Mail*, 5 May 2000, A1, A11.

McDonald, Adam D. 'Collaboration, Competition, and Coercion: Canadian Federalism and System Governance.' MA thesis, University of Waterloo, 2004.

McKillop, A.B. *The Spinster and the Prophet; Florence Deeks, H.G. Wells, and the Mystery of the Purloined Past*. Toronto: Macfarlane Walter and Ross, 2001.

McPhedran, Marilou. 'The Final Report of the Task Force on Sexual Abuse of Patients.' Toronto: College of Physicians and Surgeons of Ontario, 1991.

McVaugh, Michael R., ed. *Arnaldi de Villanova Opera Medica Omnia*, vol. 3. Barcelona: Universitat de Barcelona, 1985.

– *Medicine before the Plague: Practitioners and Their Patients in the Crown of Aragon, 1285–1345*. Cambridge: Cambridge University Press, 1993.

Merriam, Carol. 'Clinical Cures for Love in Propertius' *Elegies*.' *Scholia. Studies in Classical Antiquity* 10 (2001): 69–76.

Merskey, Harold. 'Variable Meanings for the Definition of Disease.' *Journal of Medicine and Philosophy* 11 (1986): 215–32.

Mesulam, Marek-Marsel, and Jon Perry. 'The Diagnosis of Love-Sickness: Experimental Psychophysiology with the Polygraph.' *Psychophysiology* 9 (1972): 546–51.

Mickleburgh, Rod. 'Slash, Head Bash Normal in NHL: Player.' *Globe and Mail*, 29 September 2000, A14.

Mitchinson, Wendy. *The Nature of Their Bodies: Women and Their Doctors in Victorian Canada*. Toronto: University of Toronto Press, 1991.

Mol, Annemarie. *the body multiple: ontology in medical practice*. Durham, NC: Duke University Press, 2002.

Moore, Brian. *The Doctor's Wife*. New York: Farrar, Strauss, and Giroux, 1976.

Morgan, J.P. 'What Is Codependency?' *Journal of Clinical Psychology* 47 (1991): 720–9.

Mosley, James W., Allan G. Redeker, Stephen M. Feinstone, and Robert H. Purcell. 'Multiple Hepatitis Viruses in Multiple Attacks of Acute Viral Hepatitis.' *New England Journal of Medicine* 296 (1977): 75–8.

Moss, Sandra W. 'Floating Kidneys.' In *Clio in the Clinic*, ed. Jacalyn Duffin, forthcoming.

Moynihan, Roy. 'The Making of a Disease: Female Sexual Dysfunction.' *British Medical Journal* 326 (2003): 45–7.

Mullens, Anne. 'Concern Mounts as Transfusion Medicine Loses Its Lustre.' *CMAJ* 158 (1998): 1499–502.

Nance, Brian K. 'Determining the Patient's Temperament: An Excursion into Seventeenth-Century Medical Semeiology.' *Bulletin of the History of Medicine* (1993): 417–38.

Nelkin, Dorothy, and Laurence Tancredi. *Dangerous Diagnostics: The Social Power of Biological Information.* Chicago: University of Chicago Press, 1994.

Nordahl, Thomas E., Murray B. Stein, Chawki Benkelfat, William E. Semple, Paul Andreason, Zametkin Allen, Thomas W. Uhde, and Robert M. Cohen. 'Regional Cerebral Metabolic Asymmetries Replicated in an Independent Group of Patients with Panic Disorders.' *Biological Psychiatry* 44 (1998): 998–1006.

Norwood, Robin. *Women Who Love Too Much: When You Keep Wishing and Hoping He'll Change.* New York: Pocket Books, 1985.

Oribase. 'Des amoureux.' In *Oeuvres d'Oribase en 6 volumes.* Trans. U.C. Bussemaker and C. Daremberg, 5 (1873): 413–14. Paris: Baillière, 1851–76.

Orsini, Michael. 'The Politics of Naming, Blaming, and Claiming; HIV, Hepatitis C, and the Emergence of Blood Activism in Canada.' *Canadian Journal of Political Science / Revue Canadien de Science Politique* 35 (2002): 475–98.

Osborne, Philip H. *Law of Torts.* Toronto: Irwin Law, 1999.

Ovid. 'Remedia amoris.' In *Ovid in Six Volumes.* Trans. J.H. Mozley, 2: 178–233. Cambridge, MA, and London: Harvard University Press and Heinemann, 1979.

Parsons, Vic. *Bad Blood: The Tragedy of the Canadian Tainted Blood Scandal.* Toronto: Lester Publishing, 1995.

Patrick, David M., Jane A. Buxton, Mark Bigham, and Richard G. Mathias. 'Public Health and Hepatitis C.' *Canadian Journal of Public Health* 91 Supplement 1 (2000): S18–21.

Patrick, David M., Mark W. Tyndall, Peter G. Cornelisse, Kathy Li, Chris H. Sherlock, Michael L. Rekart, Steffanie A. Strathdee, Sue L. Currie, Martin T. Schechter, and Michael V. O'Shaughnessy.

'Incidence of Hepatitis C Virus Infection among Injection Drug Users during an Outbreak of HIV Infection.' *CMAJ* 165 (2001): 889–95.

Patterson, K.D. 'Yellow Fever Epidemics and Mortality in the United States, 1693–1905.' *Social Science and Medicine* 34 (1992): 855–65.

Paulus Aegineta. 'On Lovesick Persons.' In *The Seven Books of Paulus Aegineta*. Trans. F. Adams. London: New Sydenham Society, 1844–7.

Persaud, Rajendra D. 'Erotomania.' *Contemporary Review* 256 (March 1990): 148–52.

Pert, Candace B. *Molecules of Emotion: Why You Feel the Way You Feel*. New York: Scribner, 1997.

Pert, Candace B., Henry E. Dreher, and Michael R. Ruff. 'The Psychosomatic Network: Foundations of Mind-Body Medicine.' *Alternative Therapies in Health and Medicine* 4 (1998): 30–41.

Pert, Candace B., Michael R. Ruff, Richard J. Weber, and Miles Herkenham. 'Neuropeptides and Their Receptors.' *Journal of Immunology* 135, no. 2, Supplement (1985): 820s–6s.

Pert, Candace B., and Solomon H. Snyder. 'Opiate Receptor: Demonstration in Nervous Tissue.' *Science* 179 (1973): 1011–14.

Peters, Ted. 'On the "Gay Gene": Back to Original Sin Again?' *Dialog: A Journal of Theology* 33 (1994): 30–8.

Petterson, Einar. *Amans Amanti Medicus: Das Genremotiv der ärtztliche Besuch in seinem kulturhistorischen Kontext*. Berlin: Gabr. Mann Verlag, 2000.

Picard, André. 'Family Fights to Ensure Pain Not in Vain. Blood Test, Part 2.' *Globe and Mail*, 6 September 1993, A1, A4.

– 'France Makes Example of Misdeeds. Blood Test, Part 3.' *Globe and Mail*, 7 September 1993, A1, A4.

– *The Gift of Death: Confronting Canada's Tainted-Blood Tragedy*. Toronto: HarperCollins, 1998.

– 'Hepatitis C Victims Get Little of Fund.' *Globe and Mail*, 1 April 2002, A1, A7.

– 'Lending an Arm to Save Lives, Money. Blood Test, Part 4.' *Globe and Mail*, 8 September 1993, A1, A6.

– 'RCMP Lay 32 Charges in Tainted-Blood Case.' *Globe and Mail*, fis21 November 2002, A1, A6.

- 'Restoring Faith in the Safety Net. Blood Test, Part 1.' *Globe and Mail*, 4 September 1993, A1, A6.

Pigeaud, Jackie. 'Reflections on Love-Melancholy in Robert Burton.' Trans. Faith Wallis. In *Eros and Anteros*, ed. Beecher and Ciavolella, 211–31.

Pinault, Jody Rubin. *Hippocratic Lives and Legends*. London, New York, Köln: E.J. Brill, 1992.

Pitcarnii, Archibaldi. *Opera omnia*. Lugduni Batavorum: John Arnold Langerak, 1737.

Plutarch. 'Demetrius.' In *Plutarch's Lives*. Trans. J. Langhorne and W. Langhorne, 941–66. London: J.J. Chidley, 1842.

- 'Table Talk, VIII, 9.' *Moralia with an English Translation. Loeb Classical Library*. 15 vols. Vol. 9 (1961). Trans. Edwin L. Minar, Jr, F.H. Sandback, and W.C. Helmbold, 186–203. Cambridge, MA, and London: Harvard University Press and Heinemann, 1927–69.

Pool, Judith Graham, and Angela E. Shannon. 'Production of High-Potency Concentrates of Antihemophilic Globulin in a Closed-Bag System: Assay in Vitro and in Vivo.' *New England Journal of Medicine* 273 (1965): 1443–7.

Poon, Nancy. 'Conceptual Issues in Defining Male Domestic Violence.' In *Men and Masculinities*, ed. Haddad, 245–61.

Porter, Roy. 'The Literature of Sexual Advice before 1800.' In *Sexual Knowledge, Sexual Science: The History of Attitudes to Sexuality*, ed. Roy Porter and Mikulás Teich, 134–57. Cambridge: Cambridge University Press, 1994.

Porter, Roy, and G.S. Rousseau. *Gout: The Patrician Malady*. New Haven and London: Yale University Press, 1998.

Postman, Neil. *Technopoly: The Surrender of Culture to Technology*. New York: Vintage Books, 1993.

Potter, Paul. *A Short Handbook of Hippocratic Medicine*. Quebec: Éditions du Sphinx, 1988.

- 'Some Principles of Hippocratic Nosology.' In *La maladie et les maladies dans la Collection Hippocratique; 6e Colloque International Hippocratique, 1987*, ed. Paul Potter, Gilles Maloney, and Jacques Desautels, 237–53. Quebec: Éditions du Sphinx, 1990.

Pound, Ezra, and Noel Stock. *Love Poems of Ancient Egypt*. New York: New Directions, 1976 [1962].

Prince, Alfred M. 'An Antigen Detected in the Blood during the Incubation Period of Serum Hepatitis.' *Proceedings of the National Academy of Sciences of the United States of America* 60 (1968): 814–21.

– 'Can the Blood-Transmitted Hepatitis Problem Be Solved?' *Annals of the New York Academy of Sciences* 240 (1975): 191–200.

Propertius, Sextus. *The Poems of Sextus Propertius.* Trans. J.P. McCulloch. Berkeley, Los Angeles: University of California Press, 1972.

Quadrio, Carolyn. 'Sex Gender and the Impaired Therapist.' *Australian and New Zealand Journal of Psychiatry* 26 (1992): 346–63.

Quétel, Claude. *History of Syphilis.* Trans. Judith Braddock and Brian Pike. Cambridge: Polity, 1990.

Rather, L.J. *Mind and Body in Eighteenth-Century Medicine: A Study Based on Jerome Gaub's 'De regimine mentis.'* London: The Wellcome Historical Medical Library, 1965.

Ratnoff, Oscar D. 'Why Do People Bleed?' In *Blood Pure and Eloquent: A Story of Discovery, of People, and of Ideas,* ed. Maxwell M. Wintrobe, 600–57. New York: McGraw-Hill, 1980.

Rauch, Scott L., Cary R. Savage, Nathaniel M. Alpert, D. Dougherty, A. Kendrick, T. Curran, H.D. Brown, Manzo, A.J. Fischman, and M.A. Jenike. 'Probing Striatal Function in Obsessive-Compulsive Disorder: A PET Study of Implicit Sequence Learning.' *Journal of Neuropsychiatry and Clinical Neurosciences* 9 (1997): 568–73.

Rauch, Scott L., Cary R. Savage, Nathaniel M. Alpert, Alan J. Fischman, and Michael A. Jenike. 'The Functional Neuroanatomy of Anxiety: A Study of Three Disorders Using Positron Emission Tomography and Symptom Provocation.' *Biological Psychiatry* 42 (1997): 446–52.

Rebhun, L.A. 'A Heart Too Full: The Weight of Love in Northeast Brazil.' *Journal of American Folklore* 107 (winter 1994): 167–80.

Reichl, Karl. 'Liebe als Krankheit: mittelenglische Texte.' In *Liebe als Krankheit,* ed. Stemmler, 187–220.

Reiser, Stanley Joel. *Medicine and the Reign of Technology.* Cambridge and New York: Cambridge University Press, 1979.

Remis, R.S., M.V. O'Shaughnessy, C. Tsoukas, G.H. Growe, M.T. Schechter, R.W. Palmer, and D.N. Lawrence. 'HIV Transmission to Patients with Hemophilia by Heat-Treated, Donor-Screened Factor Concentrate.' *CMAJ* 142 (1990): 1247–54.

Rice, G., C. Anderson, N. Risch, and G. Ebers. 'Male Homosexuality: Absence of Linkage to Microsatellite Markers at Xq28.' *Science* 284 (1999): 665–7.

Rice, John Steadman. *A Disease of One's Own: Psychotherapy, Addiction, and the Emergence of Co-Dependency.* New Brunswick, NJ, and London: Transaction Publishers, 1996.

Riese, Walter. *The Conception of Disease, Its History, Its Versions and Its Nature.* New York, 1953.

Riha, Ortrun. 'Subjektivität und Objektivität, Semiotik und Diagnostik. Eine Annäherung an der mittelalterlichen Krankheitsbegriff.' *Sudhoff's Archiv: Zeitschrift für Wissenschaftsgeschichte* 80 (1996): 129–49.

Ringeretz, Olaf, and Bo Zetterberg. 'Serum Hepatitis among Swedish Track Finders.' *New England Journal of Medicine* 276 (1967): 540–6.

Risse, Guenter B. 'Epidemics and Medicine: The Influence of Disease on Medical Thought and Practice.' *Bulletin of the History of Medicine* 53 (1979): 505–19.

– 'Health and Disease: History of the Concepts.' In *Encyclopedia of Bioethics,* vol. 2, ed. Warren T. Reich, 579–85. New York: Free Press, 1978.

Roberts, E.A., S.M. King, M. Fearon, and N. McGee. 'Hepatitis C in Children after Transfusion: Assessment by Look Back Studies.' *Acta Gastroenterologica Belgica* 61 (1998): 195–7.

Rohr, Rupprecht. 'Liebe als Krankheit bei den Troubadors.' In *Liebe als Krankheit,* ed. Stemmler, 139–50.

Rosario, Vernon A. *The Erotic Imagination: French Histories of Perversity.* New York and Oxford: Oxford University Press, 1997.

Rose, Geoffrey. 'Sick Individuals and Sick Populations.' *International Journal of Epidemiology* 14 (1985): 32–8.

Rosebury, Theodor. *Microbes and Morals: The Strange Story of Venereal Disease.* New York: Viking, 1971.

Rosenberg, Charles E., ed. *Explaining Epidemics and Other Studies in the History of Medicine.* Cambridge: Cambridge University Press, 1992.

– 'The Tyranny of Diagnosis: Specific Entities and Individual Experience.' *Milbank Quarterly* 80 (2002): 237–60.

– 'What Is Disease? In Memory of Oswei Temkin.' *Bulletin of the History of Medicine* 77 (2003): 491–505.

Rosenberg, Charles E., and Janet L. Golden, eds. *Framing Disease. Studies in Cultural History.* New Brunswick, NJ: Rutgers University Press, 1992.

Rosner, Fred. 'Hemophilia in Classic Rabbinic Texts.' *Journal of the History of Medicine and Allied Sciences* 49 (1994): 240–50.

Rothman, David. *Strangers at the Bedside.* New York: Basic Books, 1991.

Rowse, A.L. *Homosexuals in History: A Study of Ambivalence in Society, Literature, and the Arts.* New York: Macmillan, 1977.

Sagar, Johann Baptist Michael. *Systema morborum symptomaticum secundum classes, ordines, genera et species.* 2 vols. Vienna: J.P. Krause, 1771.

Salk, Jonas E. 'Biological Basis of Disease and Behaviour.' *Perspectives in Biology and Medicine* 5 (1962): 198–206.

Sandhu, J., J.K. Preiksaitis, P.M. Campbell, K.C. Carrière, and P.A. Hessel. 'Hepatitis C: Prevalence and Risk Factors in the Northern Alberta Dialysis Population.' *American Journal of Epidemiology* 150 (1999): 58–66.

Sappho. *If Not, Winter: Fragments of Sappho.* Trans. and ed. Anne Carson. New York: Alfred A. Knopf, 2002.

– *Songs of Sappho, Including the Recent Egyptian Discoveries.* Trans. and ed. Marion Mills Miller and David M. Robinson. Lexington, KY: Maxwelton, 1925.

Saslow, Arnold R., William M. Hammon, Russell Rule Rycheck, Eleanor Steriff, and Jessica Lewis. '"Hippie" Hepatitis: An Epidemiologic Investigation Conducted within a Population of "Street People."' *American Journal of Epidemiology* 101 (1975): 211–19.

Saunders, John. 'Letter Threatens Canada's Blood System.' *Globe and Mail,* 7 November 2001, A9.

Sauvages, François Boissier de. 'Dissertatio medica atque ludicra de amore. Utrum sit amor medicabilis herbis? [1724].' *Monspeliensis Hippocrates* 20 (summer 1963): 10–15.

– *Nosologia methodica.* 2 vols. Amstelodami: Sumptibus Fratrum de Tournes, 1768.

– *Pathologia methodica, seu de cognoscendis morbis.* Amstelodami: Sumptibus Fratrum de Tournes, 1752.

– *Pathologia methodica, seu de cognoscendis morbis,* tertia ed. Lugduni: Typis Petri de Bruyset: Fratrum de Tournes, 1759.

Sawyer, P.R., and C.R. Harrison. 'Massive Transfusion in Adults: Diagnoses, Survival, and Blood Bank Support.' *Vox Sanguinis* 58 (1990): 199–203.

Saxena, S., A.L. Brody, J.M. Schwartz, and L.R. Baxter Jr. 'Neuroimaging and Frontal-Subcortical Circuitry in Obsessive-Compulsive Disorder.' *British Journal of Psychiatry* 35, Supplement (1998): 26–37.

Saxena, S., A.L. Brody, K.M. Maidment, J.J. Dunkin., M. Colgan, S. Alborzian, M.E. Phelps, and L.R. Baxter, Jr. 'Localized Orbitofrontal and Subcortical Metabolic Changes and Predictors of Response to Paroxetine Treatment in Obsessive-Compulsive Disorder.' *Neuropsychopharmacology* 21 (1999): 683–93.

Schaef, Anne Wilson. *Co-Dependence: Misunderstood – Mistreated*. Minneapolis: Winston Press, 1986.

Schiefenhovel, Wulf. 'Perception, Expression, and Social Function of Pain: A Human Ethological View.' *Science in Context* 8 (1995): 31–46.

Schill, Thomas, Jeff Harsch, and Katie Ritter. 'Countertransference in the Movies: Effects on Beliefs about Psychiatric Treatment.' *Psychological Reports* 67 (1990): 399–402.

Schneck, J.M. 'The Love-Sick Patient in the History of Medicine.' *Journal of the History of Medicine and Allied Sciences* 12 (1957): 266–7.

Schnell, Rüdiger. *Causa amoris. Liebeskonzeption und Liebesdarstellung in der mittelalterlichen Literatur*. Bern, Munich: Francke Verlag, 1985.

Schüklenk, Udo, Edward Stein, Jacinta Kerin, and William Byne. 'The Ethics of Genetic Research on Sexual Orientation.' *Hastings Center Report* 27 (1997): 6–13.

Scull, Andrew T. *The Most Solitary of Afflictions: Madness and Society in Britain, 1700–1900*. New Haven, London: Yale University Press, 1993.

Seeff, Leonard B. 'Natural History of Hepatitis C.' *American Journal of Medicine* 107, no. 6B (1999): 10S–15S.

– 'The Natural History of Hepatitis C: A Quandary.' *Hepatology* 28 (1997): 1710–12.

Seeff, Leonard B., and Jules L. Dienstag. 'Transfusion-Associated Non-A, Non-B Hepatitis: Where Do We Go from Here?' *Gastroenterology* 95 (1988): 530–3.

Seeff, Leonard B., Richard N. Miller, Charles S. Rabkin, Zelma Bushell-Bales, Kelle D. Straley-Eeson, Bonnie L. Smoack, Lelye D. Johnson, Stephen R. Lee, and Edward L. Kaplan. '45–Year Follow-up of Hepatitis C Virus Infection in Healthy Young Adults.' *Annals of Internal Medicine* 132 (2000): 105–11.

Sennert, Daniel. *Opera*. Lugduni: Joannes Autorii Huguetan, 1656.

Sharara, A.I. 'Chronic Hepatitis C.' *Southern Medical Journal* 90 (1997): 872–7.

Shavit, Yehuda, James W. Lewis, Robert Gale, and John C. Lieberskind. 'Opioid Peptides Mediate the Suppressive Effect of Stress on Natural Killer Cell Cytotoxicity.' *Science* 223 (1984): 188–90.

Sherlock, Sheila. *Diseases of the Liver and Biliary Tract*. Oxford: Blackwell, 1968.

– 'Hepatitis C Virus: A Historical Perspective.' *Digestive Diseases and Sciences* 41 (1996): 3S–5S.

Shorter, Edward. *From Paralysis to Fatigue: A History of Psychosomatic Illness in the Modern Era*. New York and Toronto: Free Press, 1992.

Silverstein, Marc D., Albert G. Mulley, and Jules L. Dienstag. 'Should Donor Blood Be Screened for Elevated Alanine Aminotransferase Levels? A Cost-Effectiveness Analysis.' *JAMA* 252 (1984): 2839–45.

Simon, Frantisek. 'Uber den Bedeutungswandel der Suffixes "-itis" und "-oma" in der medizinischen Terminologie.' *Schriftenreihe der Geschichte der Naturwissenschaft, Technik, und Medizin* 25 (1988): 67–83.

Simon, N., J.P. Mery, C. Trepo, L. Vitvitski, and A.M. Couroucé. 'A Non-A Non-B Hepatitis Epidemic in a HB Antigen-Free Haemodialysis Unit. Demonstration of Serological Markers of Non-A Non-B Virus.' *Proceedings of the European Dialysis and Transplant Association* 17 (1980): 173–8.

Singer, Charles. 'The Visions of Hildegard of Bingen.' In *From Magic to Science: Essays on the Scientific Twilight*, 199–240. New York: Dover, [1917] 1958.

Siraisi, Nancy G. *Medieval and Early Renaissance Medicine: An Introduction to Knowledge and Practice*. Chicago: University of Chicago Press, 1990.

Skinner, Marilyn B. 'Disease Imagery in Catullus.' *Classical Philology* 82 (1987): 230–3.

Sklar, L.S., and H. Anisman. 'Stress and Coping Factors Influence Tumor Growth.' *Science* 205 (1979): 513–15.

Small, Helen. *Love's Madness. Medicine, the Novel, and Female Insanity, 1800–1865*. Oxford: Clarendon Press, 1996.

Smith, D.B., and P. Simmonds. 'Review: Molecular Epidemiology of Hepatitis C Virus.' *Journal of Gastroenterology and Hepatology* 12 (1997): 522–7.

Smith, Dale C. 'Appendicitis, Appendectomy, and the Surgeon.' *Bulletin of the History of Medicine* 70 (1996): 414–41.

Smith, Tracey D. 'Institutionalized Violence within the Medical Profession.' In *Men and Masculinities: A Critical Anthology,* ed. Haddad, 263–75.

Solomon, G.F., and R.F. Moos. 'Emotions, Immunity, and Disease.' *Archives of General Psychiatry* 11 (1964): 657.

Solomon, Michael. *The Literature of Misogyny in Medieval Spain: The 'Archipreste de Talavera' and the 'Spill.'* New York and Cambridge: Cambridge University Press, 1997.

Sontag, Susan. *Illness as Metaphor.* New York: Farrar, Strauss, and Giroux, 1977.

Soucie, J.M., R. Nuss, B. Evatt, A. Abdelhak, L. Cowan, H. Hill, M. Kolakoski, and N. Wilber. 'Mortality among Males with Hemophilia: Relations with Source of Medical Care. The Hemophilia Surveillance System Project Investigators.' *Blood* 96 (2000): 437–42.

Sournia, Jean-Charles. *A History of Alcoholism.* Trans. Nick Hindley and Gareth Stantion. Oxford: Basil Blackwell, 1990.

Spaet, Theodore H. 'Platelets: the Bood Dust.' In *Blood Pure and Eloquent: A Story of Discovery, of People, and of Ideas,* ed. Maxwell M. Wintrobe, 548–71. New York: McGraw-Hill, 1980.

Spencer, Duncan. *Love Gone Wrong: The Jean Harris Scarsdale Murder Case.* New York: Signet Book, New American Library, 1981.

Spitzer, Robert L. 'The Diagnostic Studies of Homosexuality in DSM-III: A Reformulation of the Issues.' In *Scientific Controversies,* ed. Englehardt and Caplan, 401–16.

Spitzer, Robert L., et al., eds. *DSM-IV Casebook: A Learning Companion to the Diagnostic and Statistical Manual of Mental Disorders.* Washington, DC: American Psychiatric Association, 1994.

Spurgeon, David. 'Canada's HIV Blood Inquiry Turns Poisonous.' *Nature* 384 (1997): 602.

– 'Canadian Inquiry Calls for "Safety First" Blood Agency.' *Nature* 390 (1997): 432.

- 'Canadians Sue over Hepatitis C Infection.' *British Medical Journal* 315 (1997): 330.

Stanley. P. 'Budd-Chiari Syndrome.' *Radiology* 170, no. 3, pt 1 (1989): 625–7.

Starobinski, Jean. *Histoire de la traitement de la mélancholie des origines à 1900. Acta Psychosomatica* 4. Basel: J.R. Geigy, 1960.

Starr, Donald. *Blood: An Epic History of Medicine and Commerce.* New York: Alfred A. Knopf, 1999.

Steadman, John M. 'Courtly Love as a Problem of Style.' In *Chaucer und seine Zeit. Symposium für Walter F. Schirmer,* ed. Arno Esch, 1–33. Tübingen: Max Niemyer Verlag, 1968.

Stemmler, Theo, ed. *Liebe als Krankheit. 3 Kolloquium der Forschungsstelle für Europäishe lyrik des Mittelalters.* Mannheim and Tübingen: Narr and Universität Mannheim, 1990.

Stendhal [Henri Marie Beyle]. *De l'amour/Love.* Trans. Gilbert Sale, Suzanne Sale, and Jean Stewart. London: Penguin, [1822] 1975.

Stettler, Antoinette. 'Zeichen lesen und Zeichen deuten: zur Geschichte der medizinischen Semiotick.' *Gesnerus* 44 (1987): 33–54.

Stevens, C.E., R.D. Aach, F.B. Hollinger, J.W. Mosley, W. Szmuness, R. Kahn, J. Werch, and V. Edwards. 'Hepatitis B Virus Antibody in Blood Donors and the Occurrence of Non-A, Non-B Hepatitis in Transfusion Recipients. An Analysis of the Transfusion-Transmitted Viruses Study.' *Annals of Internal Medicine* 101 (1984): 733–8.

Stevenson, Lloyd G. 'Exemplary Disease: The Typhoid Pattern.' *Journal of the History of Medicine* 37 (1982): 159–82.

Stratton, Elizabeth, Lamont Sweet, Arleen Latorrca-Walsh, and Paul R. Gully. 'Hepatitis C in Prince Edward Island: A Descriptive Review of Reported Cases, 1990–1995.' *Canadian Journal of Public Health* 88 (1997): 91–4.

Sullivan, Rosemary. *Labyrinth of Desire: A Story of Women and Romantic Obsession.* Toronto: Harper Collins Flamingo Canada, 2001.

Sydenham, Thomas. 'On Gout [Tractatus de Podagra et de Hydrope, 1683.' In *The Works of Thomas Sydenham.* 2 vols. Trans. R.G. Latham, 2: 123–62. London: Sydenham Society, 1848–50.

Tannahill, Reay. *Sex in History.* New York: Stein and Day, 1980.

Temkin, Owsei. 'The Scientific Approach to Disease: Specific Entity or

Individual Sickness.' In *The Double Face of Janus*, 441–55. Baltimore and London: Johns Hopkins University Press, [1963] 1977.

Tenner, Edward. *Why Things Bite Back: Technology and the Revenge of Unintended Consequences*. New York: Alfred A. Knopf, 1996.

Thompson, Stith. *Motif-Index of Folk-Literature*, 6 vols. Bloomington: Indiana University Press, 1955–8.

Tibbs, C.J. 'Methods of Transmission of Hepatitis C.' *Journal of Viral Hepatitis* 2 (1995): 113–19.

Tighe, Janet A. 'The Legal Art of Psychiatric Diagnosis: Searching for Reliability.' In *Framing Disease*, ed. Rosenberg and Golden, 206–28.

Trépo, Christian, and Rafael Esteban. 'Chronic HCV Infection; Public Health Threat and Emerging Consensus, Conference Held in Vienna Austria, 27 to 28 October 1995.' *Digestive Diseases and Sciences* 41, no. 12, Supplement (1996): 1S–135S.

Trivedi, Madhukar H. 'Functional Neuroanatomy of Obsessive-Compulsive Disorder.' *Journal of Clinical Psychiatry* 57 Supplement 8 (1996): 26–35.

Tsoukas, Christos, Francine Gervais, Joseph Shuster, Phil Gold, Michael O'Shaughnessy, and Marjorie Robert-Guroff. 'Association of HTLV-III Antibodies and Cellular Immune Status of Hemophiliacs.' *New England Journal of Medicine* 311 (1984): 1514–15.

Tucker, B.P. 'Deaf Culture, Cochlear Implants, and Elective Disability.' *Hastings Center Report* 28 (1998): 6–14.

U.S. Centers for Disease Control. 'Recommendations for Prevention and Control of Hepatitis C Virus (HCV) Infection and HCV-Related Chronic Disease.' *Morbidity and Mortality Weekly Reports* 47 (RR–19) (1998): 1–38.

– Hepatitis C Factsheet. http://www.cdc.gov/ncidod/diseases/hepatitis/c/fact.htm (accessed September 2004).

Utsumi, Takeshi, Etsuo Hashimoto, Yusuke Okumura, Makiko Taka-nanagi, Hiroaki Nishikawa, Mika Kigawa, Nobuchio Kumakura, and Hiroyuko Toyokawa. 'Heterosexual Activity as a Risk Factor for the Transmission of Hepatitis C Virus.' *Journal of Medical Virology* 46, no. 2 (1995): 122–5.

Van der Eijk, Philip J. 'Aristotle's Psycho-Physiological Account of the Soul-Body Relationship.' In *Psyche and Soma: Physicians and Metaphy-*

sicians on the Mind-Body Problem from Antiquity to Enlightenment, ed. John Wright and Paul Potter, 57–77. Oxford: Clarendon Oxford University Press, 2000.

Van der Poel, Cees L., H. Theo Cuyper, and Henk W. Reesink. 'Hepatitis C Six Years On.' *Lancet* 344 (1994): 1475–9.

Vidal, Fernando. 'An 18th-Century Debate about Masturbation and Lust in Young Children.' Unpublished paper, read at 'Health and the Child; Care and Culture in History,' Geneva, 13–15 September 2001.

Vollmann, Benedikt Konrad. 'Liebe als Krankheit in der weltlichen Lyrik des lateinischen Mittelalters.' In *Liebe als Krankheit*, ed. Stemmler, 105–25.

Voltaire, *Dictionnaire philosophique*. Paris: Garnier-Flammarion, [1764] 1964.

Vrettos, Athena. *Somatic Fictions: Imagining Illness in Victorian Culture*. Stanford, CA: Stanford University Press, 1995.

Wack, Mary Frances. 'From Mental Faculties to Magical Philters: The Entry of Magic into Academic Medical Writing on Lovesickness, 13th–17th Centuries.' In *Eros and Anteros*, ed. Beecher and Ciavolella, 9–31.

– 'The *Liber de heros morbo* of Johannes Afflacius and Its Implications for Medieval Love Conventions.' *Speculum* 62 (1987): 324–44

– *Lovesickness in the Middle Ages: The Viaticum and Its Commentaries*. Philadelphia: University of Pennsylvania Press, 1990.

– 'Memory and Love in Chaucer's "Troilus and Criseyde."' Thesis, Cornell University, 1982.

Walker, I.R., and J.A. Julian. 'Causes of Death in Canadians with Haemophilia 1980–1995. Association of Hemophilia Clinic Directors of Canada.' *Haemophilia* 4 (1998): 714–20.

Wallis, Faith. 'The Experience of the Book: Manuscripts, Texts, and the Role of Epistemology in Early Medieval Medicine.' In *Knowledge and the Scholarly Medical Traditions*, ed. Don Bates, 101–26. Cambridge: Cambridge University Press, 1995.

– 'Inventing Diagnosis; Theophilus's "De Urinis" in the Classroom.' *Dynamis* 20 (2000): 31–73.

– 'Signs and Senses; Diagnosis and Prognosis in Early Medieval Pulse and Urine Texts.' *Social History of Medicine* 13 (2000): 265–78.

Walzer, Richard. 'Aristotle, Galen, and Palladius on Love.' In *Greek into Arabic: Essays on Islamic Philosophy,* ed. S.M. Stern and Richard Walzer. Oriental Studies, vol. 1, 48–60. Oxford: Bruno Cassirer [1939] 1963.

Wasley, Annemarie, and Miriam J. Alter. 'Epidemiology of Hepatitis C: Geographic Differences and Temporal Trends.' *Seminars in Liver Disease* 20 (2000): 1–16.

Weiner, Herbert. 'From Simplicity to Complexity (1950–1990): The Case of Peptic Ulceration – Part I. Human Studies,' and 'Part II. Animal Studies.' *Psychosomatic Medicine* 53 (1991): 491–516 and 467–90.

West, W. Gordon. 'Boys, Recreation, and Violence: The Informal Education of Some Young Canadian Males.' In *Men and Masculinities,* ed. Haddad, 277–310.

Whatley, Mariamne H. 'The Picture of Health: How Textbook Photographs Construct Health.' In *The Ideology of Images in Educational Media: Hidden Curriculums in the Classroom,* ed. Elizabeth Ellsworth and Mariamne H. Whatley, 121–40. New York and London: Teachers College of Columbia University, 1990.

Wickelgren, Ingrid. 'Discovery of "Gay Gene" Questioned.' *Science* 284 (1999): 571.

Wilkinson, R.L. 'Yellow Fever: Ecology, Epidemiology, and Role in the Collapse of the Classic Lowland Maya Civilization.' *Medical Anthropology* 16 (1995): 269–94.

Wilson, Adrian. 'On the History of Disease-Concepts: The Case of Pleurisy.' *History of Science* 38 (2000): 271–319.

Wilson, Keither. 'Ireland Announces Compensation for Hepatitis C.' *British Medical Journal* 311 (1995): 771.

Wintrobe, Maxwell M., ed. *Blood Pure and Eloquent: A Story of Discovery, of People, and of Ideas.* New York: McGraw-Hill, 1980.

Woestman, William H. *Special Marriage Cases.* 3rd ed. Bangalore: Theological Publications, 1995.

Wolfzettel, Friedrich. 'Liebe als Krankheit in der altfranzösischen Literatur.' In *Liebe als Krankheit,* ed. Stemmler, 151–86.

World Health Organization. Factsheet. October 2000. http://www.who.int/mediacentre/factsheets/fs164/en (accessed September 2004).

World Hemophilia Federation. *Report on the Global Survey 2001*. Montreal, 2001.

Wright, Peter, and Andrew Treacher, eds. *The Problem of Medical Knowledge: Examining the Social Construction of Medicine*. Edinburgh: Edinburgh University Press, 1982.

Yee, T.T., A. Griffioen, C.A. Sabin, G. Dusheiko, and C.A. Lee. 'The Natural History of HCV in a Cohort of Haemophilic Patients Infected between 1961 and 1985.' *Gut* 47 (2000): 845–51.

Young, Allan. *The Harmony of Illusions: Inventing Post-Traumatic Stress Disorder*. Princeton, NJ: Princeton University Press, 1995.

Ziporyn, Terra. *Nameless Diseases*. New Brunswick, NJ: Rutgers University Press, 1992.

Zou, Shimian, Martin Tepper, and Antonio Giulivi. 'Current Status of Hepatitis C in Canada.' *Canadian Journal of Public Health* 91, Supplement 1 (2000): S4–S9.

Index

THE JOANNE GOODMAN LECTURES

1976
C.P. Stacey, *Mackenzie King and the Atlantic Triangle* (Toronto: Macmillan of Canada 1976)

1977
Robin W. Winks, *The Relevance of Canadian History: U.S. and Imperial Perspectives* (Toronto: Macmillan 1979)

1978
Robert Rhodes James, 'Britain in Transition'

1979
Charles Ritchie, 'Diplomacy: The Changing Scene'

1980
Kenneth A. Lockridge, *Settlement and Unsettlement in Early America: The Crisis of Political Legitimacy before the Revolution* (New York: Cambridge University Press 1981)

1981
Geoffrey Best, *Honour among Men and Nations: Transformations of an Idea* (Toronto: University of Toronto Press 1982)

1982
Carl Berger, *Science, God, and Nature in Victorian Canada* (Toronto: University of Toronto Press 1983)

1983
Alistair Horne, *The French Army and Politics, 1870–1970* (London: Macmillan 1984)

1984
William Freehling, 'Crisis United States Style: A Comparison of the American Revolutionary and Civil Wars'

1985
Desmond Morton, *Winning the Second Battle: Canadian Veterans and the Return to Civilian Life, 1915–1930* (published with Glenn Wright as joint author, Toronto: University of Toronto Press 1987)

1986
J.R. Lander, *The Limitations of the English Monarchy in the Later Middle Ages* (Toronto: University of Toronto Press 1989)

1987
Elizabeth Fox-Genovese, 'The Female Self in the Age of Bourgeois Individualism'

1988
J.L. Granatstein, *How Britain's Weakness Forced Canada into the Arms of the United States* (Toronto: University of Toronto Press 1989)

1989
Rosalind Mitchison, *Coping with Destination: Poverty and Relief in Western Europe* (Toronto: University of Toronto Press 1991)

1990
Jill Ker Conway, 'The Woman Citizen: Translatlantic Variations on a Nineteenth-Century Feminist Theme'

1991
P.B. Waite, *The Loner: Three Sketches of the Personal Life and Ideas of R.B. Bennett, 1870–1947* (Toronto: University of Toronto Press 1992)

1992
Christopher Andrew, 'The Secret Cold War: Intelligence Communities and the East-West Conflict'

1993
Daniel Kevles, 'Nature and Civilization: Environmentalism in the Frame of Time'

1994
Flora MacDonald, 'An Insider's Look at Canadian Foreign Policy Initiatives since 1957'

1955
Rodney Davenport, *Birth of the 'New' South Africa* (Toronto: University of Toronto Press 1997)

1996
Ged Martin, *Past Futures: The Impossible Necessity of History* (Toronto: University of Toronto Press 2004)

1997
Donald Akenson, *If The Irish Ran the World: Montserrat, from Slavery Onwards* (Montreal: McGill-Queen's University Press 1997)

1998
Terry Copp, *Fields of Fire: The Canadians in Normandy* (Toronto: University of Toronto Press 2003)

1999
T.C. Smout, 'The Scots at Home and Abroad 1600–1750'

2000
Jack P. Green, 'Speaking of Empire: Celebration and Disquiet in Metropolitan Analyses of the Eighteenth-Century British Empire'

2001

Jane E. Lewis, *Should We Worry about Family Change?* (Toronto: University of Toronto Press 2003)

2002

Jacalyn Duffin, *Lovers and Livers: Disease Concepts in History* (Toronto: University of Toronto Press 2005)